Sonnie's Journey

A Caregiver's Journal Through Alzheimer's

Lived and recounted by Stephen J Goetz

Compiled and written by Joan M Sciacca

2024

Sonnie's Journey

A Caregiver's Journal Through Alzheimer's

Lived and recounted by Stephen J Goetz

Compiled and written by Joan M Sciacca

Copyright © 2024 by Joan M Sciacca

First Printing: 2024
ISBN: 978-1-304-50805-8
Imprint: Lulu.com

9 781304 508058

Joan Sciacca
Joan@FinestraConsulting.com
www.FinestraConsulting.com

Hard copies and eBook can be ordered on www.LuLu.com

Dedication

For Daddy.

My hero, my inspiration, my best friend.

You taught me to greet every day with a smile.

You are my role model for finding the courage
to meet life's challenges with humor and optimism.

Table of Contents

Dedication i

Preface..1

Foreword 3

Introduction 4

Diagnosed With Alzheimer's 7

Please Take Care of Me 10

Sonnie, You Should Probably Stop Driving 14

Smoky, Her Dog...19

A Quiet Man, A Good Man. 22

Friends Are Important...26

Still Laughing And Joking 29

Doctors...32

Three Years 35

A Review, A Plan, And A Prayer 43

Into The Moderate Stage 49

The Perfect Pet...55

Losing Best Friends...63

How Important Is a Big Bathroom? VERY 72

Who Are You?.. 74

Yoooou Whoooo, Is Anyone Here?...................... 79

I'm Sick, Aren't I? 81

The Digital Picture Frame 84

I Need to Go Home NOW 91

The Last 6 Months 95

It's Been 5 Years.. 102

The Spiral Accelerates 108

Are The Physical Changes the Alzheimer's or
Something Else? 114

Her Smiles Are Gone... 120

The End of The Journey....................................... 126

Epilogue.. 131

Life Goes On 133

Preface

Shortly after Mom died, Dad asked me to write this book. I didn't even start until after more than 10 years. In the writing, I had to wade my way through lots of tears. It's time to heal.

My Dad is my hero, my inspiration, and my best friend. I would do anything for him, no matter how hard, because of the love my parents have for me and the love I have for them. If he wants a book, then he's getting a book!

I've written this book from two perspectives. My perspective: what I was feeling, and a bit more background or explanation for context. Then, Dad's email and blog entries. Dad's sections are titled Email or Blog. He always signed them "-Just me, Steve".

Dad spent time going through old pictures he wanted to include of Mom or something special to him with each blog post and for this book. While some pictures may seem a bit random, to Dad they are full of meaning.

From the day I left for college, I called Mom and Dad at least once a week. Mom did most of the talking. We could be on the phone for over an hour. After the Alzheimer's started to take hold, I spoke more and more with Dad.

Dad is like Mary Poppins: "practically perfect in every way". He can, however, be a bit stubborn. Since I tend to take after him, I like to think of it as being tenacious. He was determined to take care of Mom. He was determined that she would have the best possible life he could give her and that she would live and die at home in California.

Caregiving fulltime is not for everyone. Fortunately, Dad is caring, loving, has the patience of a saint, and is a problem solver: all qualities that he utilized in caregiving for Mom.

At the time Mom was diagnosed with Alzheimer's, I was working full time, married, and living in Arizona raising two teenage boys.

I went to California as often as I could to help Dad with caregiving. Even before Alzheimer's, Mom would always ask me, "When are you coming home?" I would tell her, "When I retire". Unfortunately, she couldn't wait for me.

Live your life NOW. You never know if you're going to get a tomorrow.

I feel like I just saw Mom yesterday. I think about her every day.

Dad and I are alike, in that, if in creating this book we can help just one person, it was worth the writing.

Daddy, here is your book. I love you.

- Joni

Foreword

Steve Goetz, from Salinas, California, cared for his wife, Sonnie, for six years after she was diagnosed with Alzheimers.

During their Journey with Alzheimer's, Steve kept family and friends updated through a series of emails, which became a touching journal that captured both frustrating and poignant moments of caregiving.

During this time and for a few years after her death, Steve was an active volunteer with the Alzheimer's Association in Monterey. He participated in Memory Walks, spoke at Alzheimer's events and wrote a blog about his experience with the disease.

This book is based on Steve's emails and blog entries.

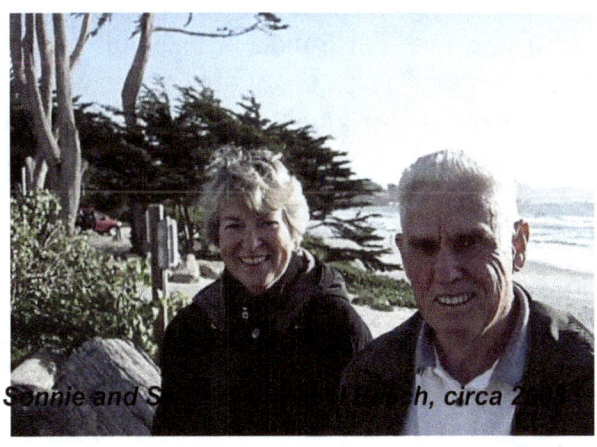

Sonnie and S........h, circa 2...

Introduction

My wife Sonnie was born and raised in a small town in Michigan. When she was 22 years old, she left Michigan for a vacation in California. When she got to Carmel, she called her parents and asked them to send her things. She wasn't going back to Michigan.

She was working as a Beautician when we met. We married eight months later. We were married for 48 years. We have two children, Jake and Joni. Sonnie was a stay-at-home mom while our kids were young and didn't return to the work force until they were in high school.

Sonnie had no major health problems until she was diagnosed with Alzheimer's disease.

My name is Steve. I'm Sonnie's husband, caregiver, lover, cook and bottle washer, but I hate to do windows. I'm 73 years old, retired after 34 years in the fire service and my health is as good as can be expected for my age.

I have some experience as a caregiver. I was the primary caregiver for my dad for two years, followed by my mom for eighteen months after he passed away.

Isn't she Beautiful! When I close my eyes, I can see her. I can't touch her, and she can't touch me, but I can see her.

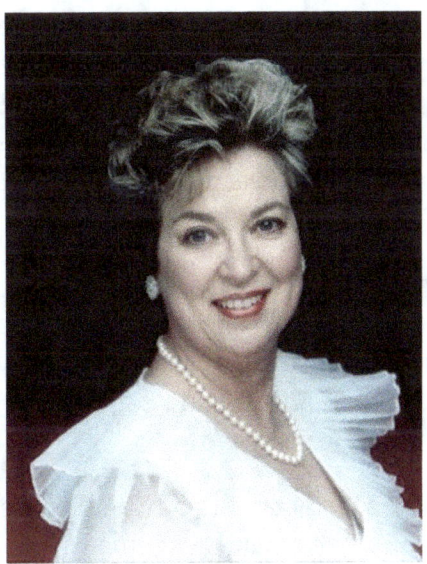

Sonnie circa 1994

It was January 17, 2003, when I first became concerned with Sonnie's memory; she couldn't remember where we kept the potholders. The problem was that the potholders were in the same drawer since we bought the house in 1972.

On September 17, 2004, Sonnie was diagnosed with Alzheimer's at Stanford University Medical Center. At that time, they understand what caused Alzheimer's.

They probably don't have enough information even today.

Three days after Sonnie was diagnosed with Alzheimer's, I met with the Monterey Alzheimer's Association. This Association became a major resource and source of support. I also started writing "Sonnie Updates", emails for friends and family. My emails were written over a six-year period and document our Journey with Alzheimer's.

Millions of people are affected by Alzheimer's. If you or someone you know has Alzheimer's or is suspected of having Alzheimer's, please share this book. I am sharing my experiences with the hope that I can help someone on their Journey with Alzheimer's.

The Alzheimer's Association has a "Caregiver" section on their website. It's full of helpful information.

At this time, it's a disease without a cure.

It's a Journey.

The challenge is how best to get through it with love and grace.

- Steve, loving husband and caregiver

Diagnosed With Alzheimer's

At first, we thought that Mom's forgetfulness was just part of menopause. I had heard that menopause can make some women forgetful. Turns out it wasn't. For a few years, we knew something was off. We never thought it would be Alzheimer's. There was no history of Alzheimer's in her family. Cancer, yes; Alzheimer's, no. It was a shock when Dad called with the news.

Alzheimer's affects the entire family. We all had to deal with our emotions as we went through the Journey with Mom. My approach was to focus on how to best help Dad.

- Joni

Email Update #1: September 18, 2004

Sonnie has been having problems with her short-term memory for the last year or so. Yesterday we returned from Stanford University Medical Center Neuroscience Clinic with the news that she is now an Alzheimer's patient. During the last few months she has been through a CT scan, MRI, MRI Angio, brain wave scan, numerous blood tests, and probably a few other tests that I've missed.

We knew that something was wrong, but you still don't like to hear the dreaded word "Alzheimer's". Alzheimer's

Disease, or dementia in any form, is not suggested in her family history. She must have gotten it from me.

The doctor has put her on some medication in an attempt to slow the progression of the disease. Now we have to strike the balance between the disease, medication side effects, and quality of life.

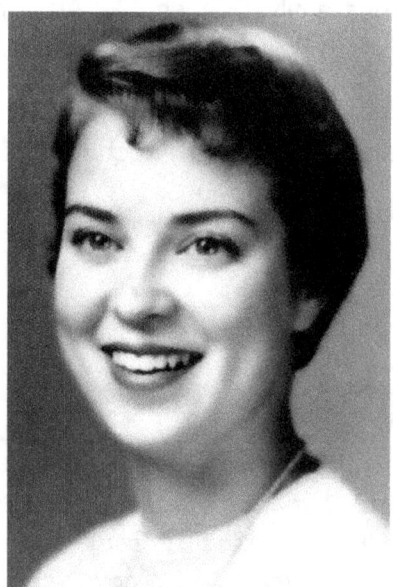

Sonnie circa 1957

Her attitude is excellent, and in a sense it's just a relief knowing what we are up against. She really likes the doctor at Stanford. He feels that with the medicine they now have to work with and the new stuff that seems to come out every day Sonnie will do fine for many years to come.

Sonnie has been playing phone tag with her brother Jack and sister Sue for the last few days. So I felt that it would be best if we did like Henry is doing for Sonnie's sister Joan and keep everyone informed by email. I have multiple email addresses for some of you and probably don't have them for others I should, but that's the way it goes.

- Just me, Steve

Please Take Care of Me

Dad is inherently a problem solver. With Alzheimer's, every day is a new problem. As the disease progresses, what worked yesterday may not work today. Dad was constantly inventing, building, and rigging things to try to make life a little more comfortable for either or both.

He is also a change agent. He wants to share his experiences, suggestions, and tips on what he did or, in hindsight, what he could have done to make things easier.

Dad is no different from the rest of us. He's sometimes plagued with survivors' guilt, that he should have done more, he should have done things differently, he should have been a better husband, he should have been a better father, he should have... and the list goes on. I keep telling him to stop thinking about all the things he should have done. No one could have done better. He went above and beyond in so many large and small ways. All anyone can do is his or her best, and he certainly did that each and every day.

He wants to share his experiences in the hope that it will assist others.

While Mom was able, I would chat with her on the phone, then switch over to Dad. Over the weeks and months, my conversations with Mom became shorter. When she was no longer able to follow the thread of the conversation, she would hand the phone over to Dad.

Every day presented a new problem to solve.

I take after Dad in the problem-solving department. Our conversations tended to be about everyday challenges, what he did and what he might try next. We did a lot of brainstorming on the phone. Staying focused on what he or I could do, and letting go of what we couldn't do, or change, was one of our coping strategies.

- Joni

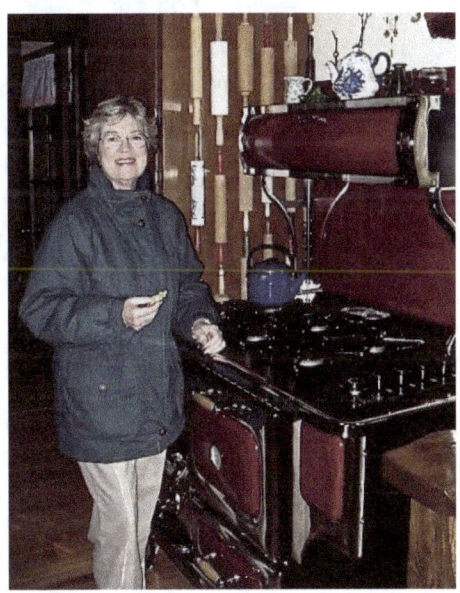

Sonnie in our cabin circa 2005

<u>Blog entry</u>

Alzheimer's is a Journey that changed our lives.

As we were driving home from Stanford after Sonnie was diagnosed with Alzheimer's, she asked me to take care of her but not to tell her what might happen in the future. I kept that promise.

Alzheimer's or dementia, in any form, was not suggested in her family history. Her first question to the doctor was, "What did I do to get it?" His answer was, "You didn't do anything to get it".

Today, the Alzheimer's Association offers a program for people in the early stages of the disease. The class sounds pretty neat. I don't think it was available when we started our Journey or I'm sure we would have attended. It's hosted by a professional and is interactive in a way that should make everyone comfortable. The people that have dementia and the person(s) that are traveling with them on their Journey will receive a roadmap to help guide them along the way.

It's important that you know that Sonnie was easy to take care of most of the time. As we travel through this Journey you will read about the traumatic times, as well as the good and fun times.

We spent a lot of time at the beach; she loved the ocean. We danced in the living room. We walked around the neighborhood and visited with our neighbors. But most of the time, we just sat and talked, held hands, and listened to music.

Alzheimer's can last anywhere from a few years to over 20. No one can tell you how long your Journey will be. All you can do is take one day at a time and make the most of it.

Find the joy in the little things.

- Just me, Steve

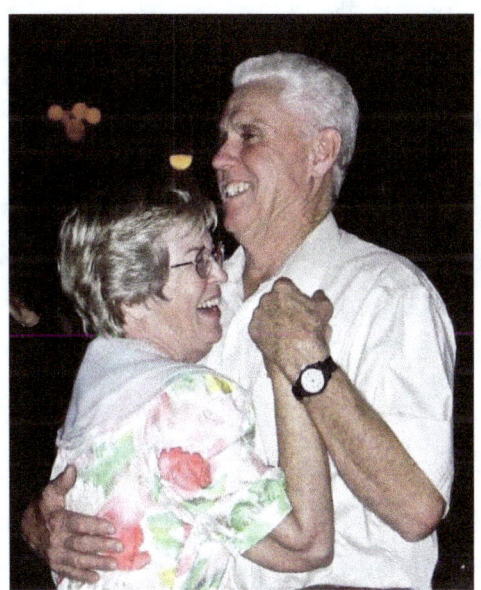

Sonnie and Steve dancing at their granddaughter's wedding, circa 2007

Sonnie, You Should Probably Stop Driving

Mom went through a denial phase.

She did her best to maintain a semblance of normalcy. She didn't want her life to change.

Mom did a good job of hiding things from Dad, for a while. I guess that's a byproduct of not wanting to know anything about the disease, or what to expect. She just kept on as best she could.

She always wanted to help and do her part. As the disease progressed, doing her part changed, as well. Dad always tried to find things that she could do to maintain some sense of independence.

Driving was the first big change.

- Joni

Email Update #2: September 17, 2005

When we first met the doctor at Stanford, he gave Sonnie a thorough checkup. He asked a series of questions and presented some problem-solving situations.

The questions and problems were used as a baseline for all future visits. Near the end of our session, after we were told that some of the indicators pointed toward Alzheimer's disease, he told Sonnie, "Sondra, you should probably stop driving."

I remember that she took a deep breath and said,

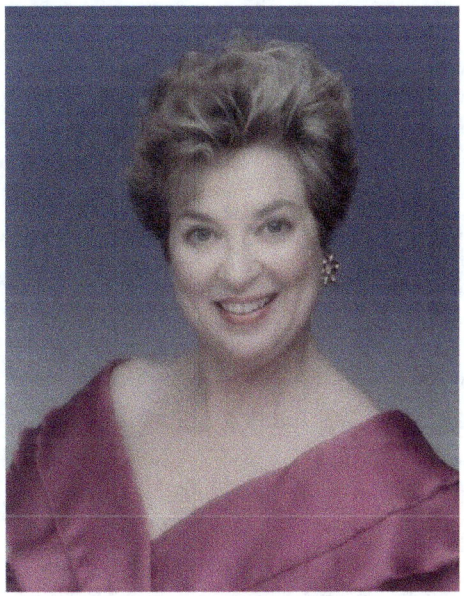

Sonnie circa 1994

"Thank God, it was getting to where I was afraid, I wouldn't find my way home." The doctor told us that he was required to notify DMV and advise them of her condition.

She was happy that she didn't have to drive. I was surprised because I didn't even realize she was having a problem driving.

I enrolled Sonnie with MedicAlert and Alzheimer's Patient's Safe Return. It's one of those things that doesn't cost much and took a load off my shoulders. I bought a Car Seatbelt Emergency ID Pocket. It's red and fits over the seatbelt. If there is an accident, the emergency personnel will have the information they need to give her the proper assistance.

Many of us that are caring for someone who has a disability (not only Alzheimer's) are not as young as we used to be (for that matter, none of us are as young as we used to be).

It has been one year since Sonnie was told that she has Alzheimer's disease, so this is as good a time as any to give everyone an update.

Sonnie is doing very well. She is happy and we joke around. We laugh a lot and spend most of our time together. I don't think she feels as good as she lets on, probably because of her medicine and the side effects. On our last trip to Stanford University Medical Center our doctor said that there is very little change in her condition from when he first saw her last September. I can tell that there is a little change, but she has a good attitude and is holding up well.

Sonnie doesn't drive the car anymore (because of the medicine) and hasn't for the past year. She tries to cook our meals but has difficulty putting a dinner together; her memory just won't put things in the right order. I help when I can, and we make a good team.

Housework must be deeply ingrained in her; our home always looks nice. We have two homes now, one in Salinas and our cabin in Big Sur. Over the last year we remodeled our cabin to her specifications, and it really looks good; we spend about half of our time there.

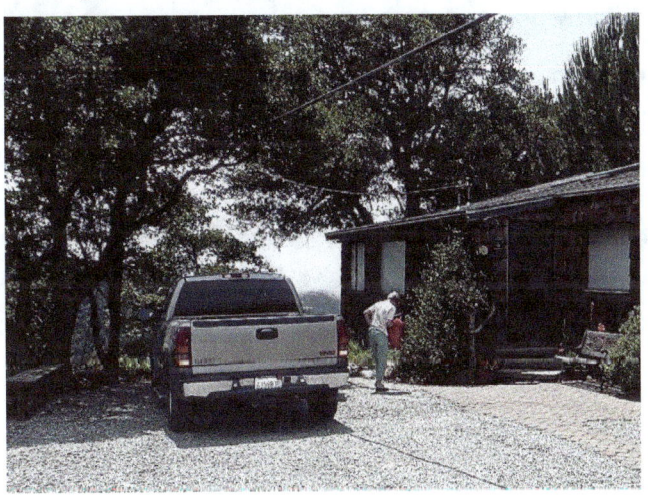

Sonnie walking into our cabin circa 2009

Sonnie's Stanford Medical Center Doctor asked if we would be interested in helping with an experiment for detecting Alzheimer's disease in its very early stages. We agreed. Although the experiment won't help Sonnie, it may help someone else down the road. We were both given MRIs. I'm not sure what the next step is, but we are ready.

We have another cliff-hanger facing us. During recent tests a spot on her liver was found. Last week she had a CT scan, and the spot was confirmed. The Doctor retrieved data on some tests that were taken in the mid 1990s to compare. If the spot was on that film, he feels we're safe, otherwise she would have been dead by now. If there is no spot on the old test, well, we'll worry about that when and if the time comes.

We think and talk about all our friends and extended family often; from the time when Sonnie was a child, to the day we met. We love all of you. If you have some time, drop Sonnie a card or letter, maybe give her a call. If she cries, it's because she is so happy that you called. If she laughs, it's because she is so happy that you called.

Sonnie will be 66 on September 14. Please send a card. She loves to get cards in the mail.

- Just me, Steve

Smoky, Her Dog

Animals can make a huge difference in our lives. Dogs give us unconditional love, especially when they are warm and cuddly. They are a living being we can cling to in times of great stress and uncertainty. They can bring us peace.

"Emotional support animals provide emotional support simply by being there for their handlers. They provide unconditional love, and just spending time with a loyal companion can really make someone who suffers from a mental disorder feel better. They also create a sense of purpose and responsibility."
www.servicedogcertifications.org

Emotional Support Benefits from Dogs
- Companionship.
- Reduced Levels of Stress. Spending time with your pet is known to lower stress levels.
- Lessens Isolation. Having a pet lessens one's isolation.
- Reduces Anxiety.
- Keep You Distracted. Pets keep your mind off issues that might be plaguing you.[1]

Smoky was Mom's dog. They were perfect for each other. He was an older dog who was happy to be carried around. He was greatly loved and gave that and more in return.

-   Joni

---

[1] Information sourced from therapypet.org

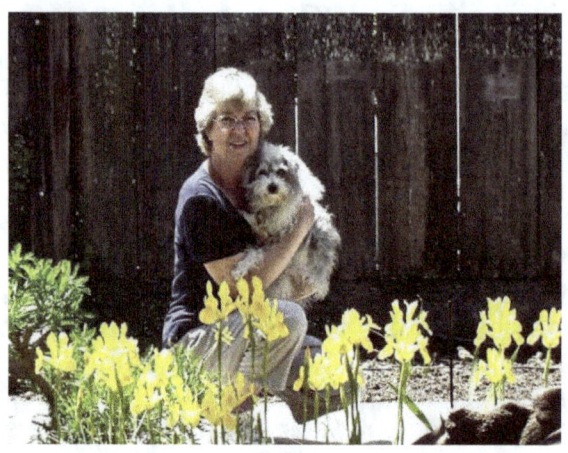

Sonnie and Smoky circa 2006

<u>Blog entry</u>

Our kids Jake and Joni and their families have been great; they are always doing stuff for us. The latest example is a dog for Sonnie.

Almost a year after Sonnie was told that she had Alzheimer's, Jake's wife Cheryl brought home a little old Border Terrier mix that had wandered into the fire station where she worked.

The dog was nearly dead. It was flea infested, sick, skinny, and filthy. They cleaned it up, took it to the Veterinarian, had it fixed up, and brought it home. Jake and Cheryl live about 100 yards or so from our cabin. Sonnie and I were at our cabin when Jake and Cheryl brought the dog so we could see it. As soon as Sonnie saw that little dog, she fell in love with it. I think it was love at first sight for both of them. She immediately said, "Can I have it?" Cheryl looked at me, and Sonnie got her dog. She held the dog to her body just as you would a baby and talked to it as you would your child.

Joni and her family came up with a list of names and from that list Sonnie chose the name Smoky.

As I look back now, I think that if Sonnie had had to choose between me and Smoky, I would have lost! Smoky came into her life at exactly the right time. She would carry Smoky everywhere and he loved it. He was old, and his last three years were the best years of his life.

I guess what I'm trying to say is – if you don't have a pet or something that the person you are caring for can cling to, talk to, and love, you might want to start looking for one.

You won't be too far into your Journey before you find your social life dropping off to almost nothing.

Alzheimer's effects everyone. Your friends and family don't know what to do or how to help. And Sonnie was changing too. Some people she would accept in her life while others she rejected. Having that dog gave her something soft to hold and love. It was perfect for her, those first few years.

- Just me, Steve

A Quiet Man, A Good Man.

Dad was determined to keep Mom at home. He was also very practical. He did check out a few care facilities for Alzheimer's and memory patients. Sometimes he would go alone when someone could care for Mom and other times, he would take Mom to see how she would react. It was like trying to put a cat into a bucket of water. She would put on the brakes and refuse to enter. I went with him a few times to see for myself. I can certainly understand why Mom wouldn't enter. Even the best places give off a sad and depressing vibe.

He did make arrangements for her should anything happen to him. He had a written care plan and had a facility selected. The plan was that, should anything happen to Dad, Mom would be taken care of until I could get there and make arrangements to bring her to Arizona. I had selected a place near me just in case. Thankfully, none of his planning was required.

Each caregiver finds his or her own way on the Journey. It's important to have a support network and examples of people who are doing things the same way you want to do it. Dad wanted to keep Mom at home. He was determined that Mom would die at home. Some people can manage it and others can't. It doesn't make it right or wrong, good, or bad. It just is the way it is and it's important for a caregiver to have examples that fit his or her chosen path. We all have a similar Journey, it's the paths that vary.

- Joni

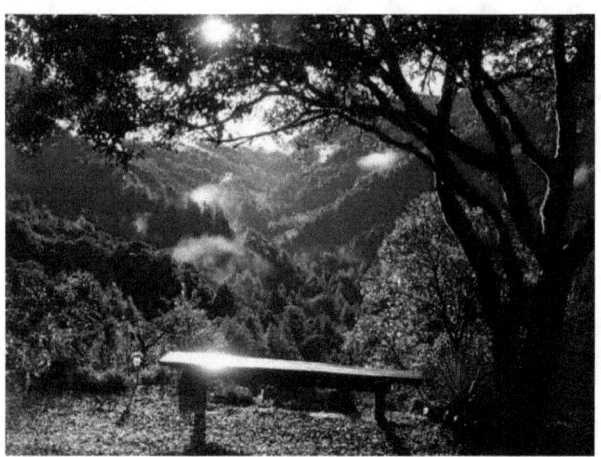

The view from our cabin, circa 2010

<u>Blog entry</u>

I want to take a step back from Sonnie's Journey and pay tribute to a man from the Alzheimer's support group that I attended for about a year.

I'll call this man "Cotton".

The Journey he and his wife took paralleled the Journey Sonnie and I were on. Cotton's a quiet man and a good man. The love he shared with his wife was over the top – unequalled.

Just one example. All people that have Alzheimer's, at one point or another, get lonely, and sometimes, just sometimes, they need companionship, friendship and just the closeness of being around other people. Not too many months ago Cotton made arrangements for his wife to stay at a home that cares for those with dementia. Yet he would be there to assist her with her breakfast, lunch, and dinner. I bet he was there when she would retire for the night, too. His hope was that she would find comfort being around other people. She didn't.

Only a few months after that, he determined what she needed was to be back home. He needed her back home.

Now those of you reading this must realize that many of us caring for our wives or husbands are not spring chickens anymore and the challenges are many. Cotton's wife passed away a little more than a month after Sonnie's Journey ended. Even though we only saw each other once a month and for only a year, I'm proud to call him a friend – a good friend.

Cotton is a quiet man and a good man.

- Just me, Steve

Friends Are Important

Everyone is affected by Alzheimer's disease. Most people don't know what to do or how to interact.

What can you say?

Friends slowly evaporate.

There are a few hearty souls who hang in there to the end. Their courage and love are amazing.

So, what can you do? How can you help? You've only to ask.

The best gift is time. Give of your time. Visit while you can.

- Joni

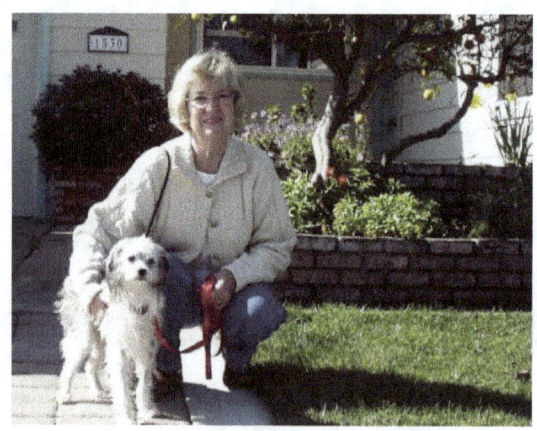

Sonnie and Smoky circa 2006

Good news! There's nothing wrong with Sonnie's liver.

It's been two years since Sonnie was told that she has Alzheimer's disease. The doctor at Stanford Medical Center says that she is still in the mild stages of the disease and answers the baseline questions like her first visit.

At home I can see a slow decline, but we just take one day at a time.

We have her medicine adjusted to where she feels a lot better and that is a big help.

It only took me about two months to get her excused from jury duty and they are even going to let me off. I have to check-in every year though.

Sonnie is registered with the Alzheimer's Association and has a necklace with her name and phone number on it. She will soon have a transmitter on her wrist. It looks like a watch and the sheriff's rescue team have a receiver that should be able to locate her in a matter of minutes. Well, they'll either locate her or the table next to the bed when I forget to put it on her.

Smoky, her dog! Smoky is the best thing that ever happened to her (after me of course). She eats, sleeps, and lives for Smoky.

Sonnie was scheduled to have a reunion with Susan, a good friend from high school in July. Susan invited us to visit her at her home in Southern California, but I don't think it is going to happen. Mainly because of the fear factor. Sonnie has pretty much lost her self-confidence and that keeps us close to home.

Sonnie turns 68 on September 14 and she is still the most beautiful woman I know.

Call or write when you can; she loves to hear from her friends. If there is anything you want her to remember, have her write it down or talk to me.

- Just me, Steve

Still Laughing And Joking

While Mom was in the mild stages of Alzheimer's disease, life continued to move along. Dad kept a positive outlook on life. He did his best to care for and entertain Mom.

They went everywhere together.

He created photo albums to help her remember things.

They spent time walking and hanging out at the beach.

The love they shared was incredible. They had the kind of love we all hope to find one day.

I continued to travel to California as often as I could. I wanted to spend time with Mom, help, and make sure Dad wasn't just putting a happy spin on things to spare me from the truth of the situation.

- Joni

Email Update #4: March 14, 2007

It has been over two and a half years since Sonnie was told that she has Alzheimer's disease, so here is a six-month update. She is doing very well, she's happy, we laugh and joke around a lot and spend most of our time together. She's not feeling as good as she lets on, and the doctor continues to work with her medicine.

On our February visit to Stanford, the doctor said that things still look good, very little change from our September visit.

I can see a change, but she still has a good attitude and is holding up well.

There are three stages to Alzheimer's disease: mild, moderate, and late. Sonnie is in the mild stage and probably approaching the moderate stage. The disease can last as long as twenty years or as few as three. The average is around nine years.

Sonnie is young as far as Alzheimer's patients go and has excellent doctors. We are hoping that a new

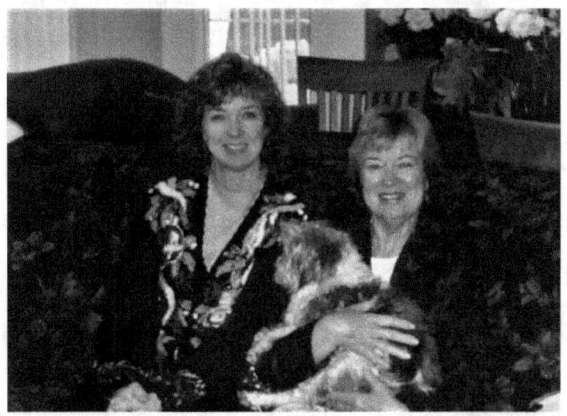

Joni, Sonnie and Smoky circa December 2006

medicine is developed to reverse the damage and give her a good quality of life.

Smoky, her dog, is still the best thing that has happened for Sonnie. She talks to him, feeds him by hand and he sleeps on our bed. Smoky allows me to leave the house for a few hours without having to worry (maybe a little) while I'm gone.

Call or write when you can. Talking with her friends or getting mail is great for her morale.

- Just me, Steve

Doctors

While doing whatever I could to help Dad, I was also very focused on his health. He was in great shape, and I wanted to keep him that way. He was so focused on Mom that I worried he wouldn't take good care of himself, physically or mentally.

The caregiver needs at least as much attention as the patient.

I felt that my job was to worry about Dad; to keep an eye on him to make sure he didn't push himself to a breaking point.

Caregiving is like taking an airplane ride. Put on your oxygen mask before assisting others. A Caregiver who gives so much that they don't have anything left for themselves will end up in distress and unable to provide care for anyone else.

I was slowly losing Mom. I didn't want to lose Dad in the process.

I was lucky. Their doctors kept on eye on both.

- Joni

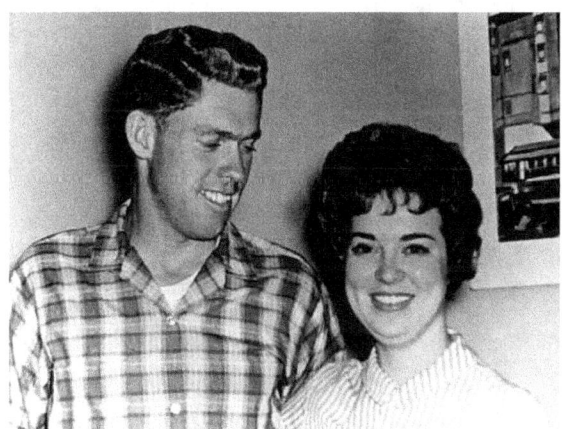

Steve and Sonnie circa 1962

Blog entry

We were fortunate to have excellent doctors through our Journey. While listening to others at different support group meetings, I found that many caregivers are not happy with their doctors. When a doctor's name is mentioned, others will say "Oh, don't go to him, he doesn't understand Alzheimer's".

Probably the best way to find a doctor who works well with a person who has Alzheimer's is through word of mouth. Join a support group or visit a couple to ask questions. If you don't have a doctor, the Alzheimer's Association in your area may be able to offer some suggestions.

It was one of Sonnie's doctors who got us into Stanford for her testing and diagnosis. His mother had

Alzheimer's. He recognized the symptoms and was extremely helpful and supportive.

Alzheimer's is one of those diseases where you really can't comprehend the challenges for both patient and caregiver until you are faced with them.

- Just Me, Steve

Three Years

At three years, Mom was slowly slipping away. I had occasional glimpses of my mom, but she was disappearing. I spent more and more time on the phone with Dad. He tried to shield me during our calls. I got my details the same as everyone else, through his email updates or visits when I could see for myself.

While we were still able, I tried to get Mom and Dad out of the house and their daily routine. We did manage a trip to Redding to visit their long-time best friends. Lois had been diagnosed with Leukemia. Ben and Lois were like second parents to me. I wanted to see them too. So, we contacted Dad's cousin in the area, and he offered to let us use his cabin on Shasta Lake. I rented a minivan, loaded up Mom, Dad, and my two sons, and off we went. The trip went well. I was so glad we had the opportunity.

We tried one other trip. I wanted Mom and Dad to come out to Arizona for a visit. I told Dad that it would be no problem. There was a direct flight from Monterey to Phoenix. He and Mom could get on the airplane in Monterey, which is a tiny airport, and just under 2 hours they would get off in Phoenix. I would tell the airline that I'm meeting my parents, that Mom has Alzheimer's, and I could get a pass to meet them at the gate.

I was at my desk at work about halfway into what should have been their flight when I got a call from Dad. They were in San Diego.

WHAT? That wasn't the plan!

He said their flight was canceled and they were able to grab a flight to San Diego with a connection to Phoenix. Here's the flight number and time we arrive. Bye - got to run to catch our flight to Phoenix.

Crap!

Mom did great. The only issue was when she had to use the toilet. Dad let her go into the ladies' room while he rushed into the men's room, planning to catch her on the way out. As he came out of the men's room, he caught a glimpse of her wandering down the concourse. He quickly caught up to her. It was a close call, but disaster averted.

That was the last time they tried to travel. I think of that event every time I see a family toilet at the airport.

- Joni

Email Update #5: August 27, 2007

On August 10th, in the morning, Sonnie had her annual physical and lab work completed. The only problem the doctor found is that her cholesterol is high at 248. We are going to try dieting and exercise first and in six months she will have another blood test. We're not big on fish. So, if you have any fish recipes that don't taste like fish, send them to us.

How many ways can you cook chicken or turkey?

In the afternoon of August 10th, we met with her doctor at the Stanford Medical Center. It has almost been three years since she was diagnosed with Alzheimer's. The test that they gave Sonnie was pretty much the same test that they gave her on her first visit. In that way the doctor can evaluate the progression of the disease.

She is still in the mild stage.

Sonnie may qualify for an experimental program at University of California, San Francisco (UCSF). The drug being tested is in stage three of four before approval is considered. I'll give you more information if we qualify; as of today, we have not been contacted.

Here are some comments on Sonnie's condition:

1)   Physically she looks the same. A very beautiful woman.
2)   She can only understand one thought at a time and only for a short period. So, if I say, "Would you feed the dog and give him some water," she may give him water, or she may feed him. She can't do both.
3)   She can't remember our married history.

4)   There have been times when she was unable to remember we have a daughter, Joni. She could remember her sister Joan but not our daughter. When she hears our daughter's voice or sees her, no problem.

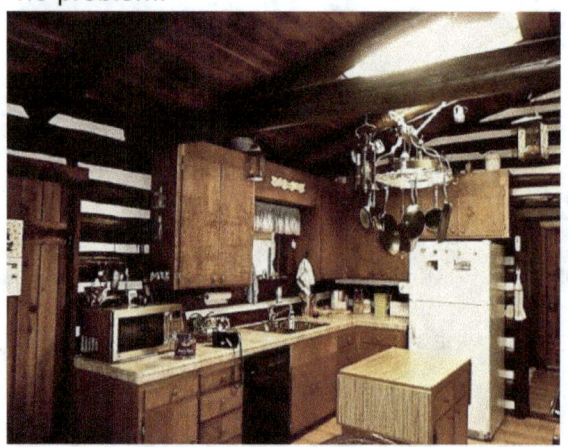

Steve and Sonnie's log cabin circa 2007

5)   She can't picture in her mind what our house looks like inside or out when we are away. The same thing with the cabin. Right now, we are picking out tile for a new countertop at the cabin. I must take pictures of the existing countertop and background so she will know what I am talking about. I showed them to her when we were in the store. I want to involve her in as much "stuff" as I can.

6)   Mornings are not good for Sonnie. For whatever reason she just doesn't feel well. It reminds me of

when she had morning sickness while pregnant with the kids.

7) Sending Christmas cards is a thing of the past. Last year some of you may have received one, two or even three, while others didn't receive any. This year I will send a note by email.

8) The dishes in the dishwasher may get washed up to three times with or without soap. She wants to do her share of whatever she thinks she can do, and I like clean dishes so it's all good.

9) Washing clothes is a little different. She and I both forget to take the Kleenex out of her pants pockets, and we are surprised by how much Kleenex she can get in her pockets.

10) Joni was here in June and she and Sonnie went through her closet and arranged it so Sonnie's choices on what to wear are limited. It takes her a long time to get dressed. She gets dressed then redressed and redressed again.

11) One time Sonnie had on two bras (both outside her blouse).

12) Once she put on six pairs of socks. Six is the record. Often, she has two pairs on and most of the time the socks don't match.

13) Her biggest problem now is saying what she wants to say. She can't think of a word to complete her idea, and in most cases, she will just say, "forget it, it wasn't important anyway".

14) Have you ever brushed your teeth with Desitin? She almost did, but she is good at coming to me when she is not sure about something.

15) Making a Peanut butter and jelly sandwich sounds pretty simple, right? Wrong! I was putting a jigsaw puzzle together in the front room and Sonnie was hungry, so I suggested a peanut butter sandwich. Well, she wanted to make it if I could help her find the stuff. I put a paper napkin on the counter, two slices of bread, and the peanut butter and jam, plus a butter knife to spread everything around, and went back to my puzzle. A short time later, here comes Sonnie with a folded paper towel, peanut butter and jam spread on the fold, and then folded in half again. No bread. She looked at me and looked at the sandwich and we both started to laugh. It was great! I know she felt bad, but I was so happy that she could laugh about it.

That will give you an idea of what she is going through and what a learning process it is for me.

I just found out a month or so ago that if she doesn't wear her earrings, the holes in her ears will close (guess what).

All in all, she is doing pretty good. She seems to be happy most of the time.

Smoky (her dog) is her whole life. She eats, sleeps, and lives for Smoky.

Sonnie turns 68 on September 14th. If you get a chance, send her a card, or give her a call. She loves to get mail and talk on the phone. But again – if there is anything that you want her to remember, have her write it down or talk to me.

I'll send out another update if anything exciting happens, otherwise our next appointment at Stanford is in April of 2008.

PS: Several of you have asked how I am doing. Everything is good with me. Sonnie and I get along great. I can still go to Home Depot by myself, cut wood, work on the water system and in the garden. The retired Fire Chiefs have a luncheon once a month where we sit around and all talk at once. None of us can hear very well, but we smile and laugh and talk about fires we fought, friends that are gone, enlarged prostates, erectile dysfunction, and whatever else old men talk about.

- Just Me, Steve

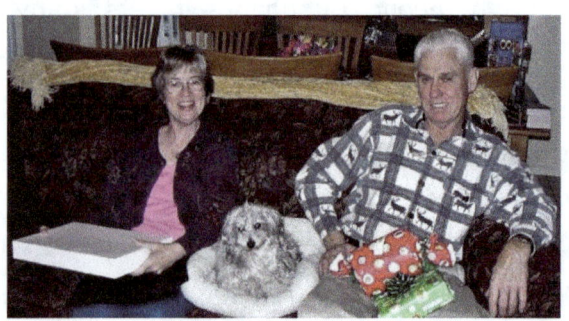

Sonnie, Smoky and Steve circa December 2006

A Review, A Plan, And A Prayer

Mom had slowly slid into the next phase of Alzheimer's and was now picking up speed.

Dad had always had what seemed like boundless energy, optimism, and courage to face what life put in front of him.

Now he was starting to wear down, and thankfully he had the self-awareness and presence of mind to add that to his list of problems to solve.

He asked me to help him put together a caregiver plan. He wanted to reach out to friends and family to create a support network around Mom. We found some examples of Care Plans and tailored one for Mom. He reached out to everyone he thought might be willing to provide help and occasional support and consolidated the responses into Mom's Care Plan.

Smart man!

- Joni

Email Update #6: May 05, 2008

Sonnie has advanced to the moderate stage or stage two of three for Alzheimer's patients.

I don't leave her alone for any length of time. I've upgraded our cell phones to a chaperone system. Sonnie's cell phone is in the silent mode in her pocket and if we get separated, I can locate her using GPS. It should get me close to her, anyway.

Sonnie hasn't driven the car since 2004, and we work pretty much as a team on everything we do.

Cooking has not been one of her high points for the last few years (for that matter, it isn't one of mine either). I'm gaining weight and she is losing it. Last month she was down to 100 pounds. As of this morning, I have her back to 103 pounds.

She's doing really well because we can laugh at so many of things that happen. I told you about the time she almost brushed her teeth with Desitin. Well, last month she came into the kitchen with blue toothpaste all through her hair wondering what went wrong. I must help her wash her hair and brush her teeth. I even lay her clothes out on the bed, but that doesn't mean that she puts them on without changing into two or three other outfits.

My last update was in August 2007, and it gave you several examples of her condition. Since then, her Alzheimer's has accelerated, and her condition has deteriorated.

The last eight months haven't been kind to us or some of our friends. One of our very best long-time friends, Lois, passed away the morning after Thanksgiving from leukemia. Lois and Ben have been close, close friends forever. Ben was the best man at our wedding. He and I date back to the Neanderthal days. I remember when Ben and Lois were married and moved into their first cave. It's not good to lose your friends.

On August 7, 2007, we lost another of my best friends, Ron, to a brain tumor. Ron and Ginger had the world by the tail before Ron got sick. The world was their playground. Now, Ben and Ginger are playing a big part in my life. They are role models for me in how to be a caregiver. If I can do half as good at caregiving for Sonnie as Ben did for Lois and Ginger did for Ron, I'll be happy.

We had to have Smoky put to sleep in early January. He just got too old, too blind, and had trouble standing up. We had him cremated and now he is at rest in a little box on our desk next to a picture of him and Sonnie. There are times that Sonnie thinks he is still here. She will ask, "Did you feed the dog?" "Where is the dog?" She has trouble remembering the name Smoky.

She has trouble remembering any names, in fact. Everyone is referred to as "the people", or "that girl" and so on. A couple days ago, Jake (our son) and I were cutting down dead trees from the Sudden Oak Death problem on the Big Sur coast. Sonnie was there with us watching the trees fall. I went down to talk to her for a few minutes to see how things were going. After a while she looked over at our son and said, "That man is sure a good worker. I bet that his mother is proud of him."

Sonnie only remembers the names of a few people consistently, and they are from her childhood. The lucky ones are Patty, Prudy and Suzan. The rest of us she can remember on her good days, sometimes. Jim and Prudy came out from Michigan to visit for a week in early January. We had a great time. I'm glad that they came out when they did because now, I think they would see a difference in Sonnie's speech.

I will be taking classes from the Alzheimer's Association on becoming a "Savvy Caregiver". Wish me luck or maybe this is where part of the Prayer should come in. A good place to get any information on Alzheimer's is www.alz.org. You can even donate!

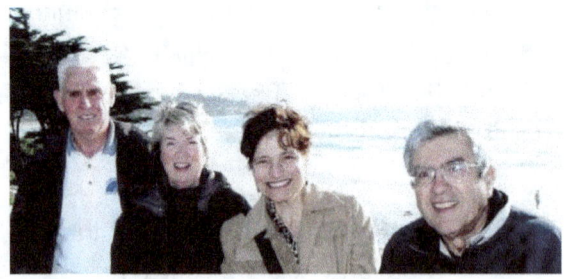

From left to right:
Steve, Sonnie, JoAnn and Joe circa 2008

Sonnie's Journey

Sonnie and I are really lucky to have friends like Joe and JoAnn. We go out to dinner once or twice a month, they drive us to some of our appointments, or do things with Sonnie when I can't.

And that leads me to "The Plan".

Recently, I found out that I am no longer faster than a speeding bullet, nor can I jump tall buildings in a single bound. Those days are gone forever, and I will need help, on occasion, with watching over Sonnie.

Our daughter Joni and I put together Sonnie's Care Plan knowing that in the days ahead there will be times that I will need YOU, or at least some of you (hopefully only a few of you), to stand in if I'm sick or need surgery or just a few hours of sleep. Somewhere down the road I know I will need to work with The Alliance on Aging and use resources available on a professional level, but right now I would prefer that our friends and relatives give us a hand. Sonnie will be a lot more comfortable and so will I.

I'll send you The Plan. Please look it over and make any comments or additions you think might help. Even if you can't physically help, your ideas will.

So! What will you do when the phone rings at 3 in the morning and it's me calling for help?

- Just Me, Steve

	1	2	3
Name			
Home Phone			
Cell Phone			
Cell Phone			
Work Phone			
Work Phone			
Address			
City, State & Zip			
email			
other contact info			
other contact info			

Please check those activities which you would be willing to perform:

Short Term Care:

1-2 hours			
2-4 hours			
4-6 hours			
6-8 hours			
1-8 hours			
1-10 hours			
10-12 hours			
Overnight			

Helpful Tasks:

Dr. Appointments			
Drivng Errands			
Cook meals			

Other ideas where you could help:

Example Care Plan created for Sonnie

Sonnie's Journey

Into The Moderate Stage

In the moderate stage, Mom's condition started to deteriorate faster, and Dad's updates increased in frequency.

Public restrooms continued to be a problem. Dad eventually got a small personal portable travel toilet and a screen he could set up next to his pickup truck to avoid the whole public restroom issue. Good idea.

Mom's ability to communicate was nearly gone.

She continued to want to help whenever she could.

During one of my visits, we decided to make cookies. I got out the recipe and all the ingredients. I spent close to an hour slowly and patiently reading the recipe to Mom and helping her measure and dump. She was more interested in reading the recipe than in making the cookies, so that's where we spent our time.

- Joni

Email Update #7: September 3, 2008

It's been four years now since the start of our Journey and the last couple of updates have been as much for me as they have been for you. I told myself that I would probably stop sending updates when Sonnie reached the middle (moderate) stage of the disease. She is now close to a year into the moderate stage.

I'll continue to write down notes of her Journey and send them to those that would like to ride along with us. I must tell you though that the rest of the trip will be depressing. If you would like to continue to receive updates, let me know. If I don't hear from you, I will remove you from my email distribution and won't send further updates. I understand that you would rather remember Sonnie as she was and not as she is going to become.

Her birthday is coming up on September 14th, and what you can do is send her a birthday card. She loves mail. She still can talk on the phone but doesn't understand it very well. I don't know, but for whatever reason she can talk to her brother Jack and sister Sue and have a reasonable conversation. The rest of us get the limited version.

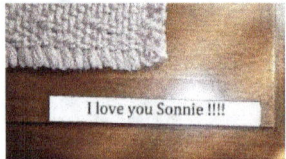 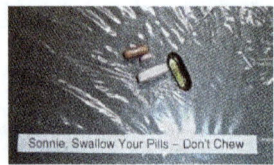

Examples of labels left around the house, circa 2008

The moderate stage can last anywhere from two to ten years, and we will see changes in how she acts, walks, finds her way around the house, and deals with noises and crowds.

In the early stage I put Post-It notes around the house to help her get through the day. Because of my essential tremors, though, my handwriting is nearly unreadable. Joni suggested that I get a labeling machine so Sonnie could read the notes. I did and it helped, for a while.

I find that whatever I do, I don't do it for long. Now I am picking up the labels as they are no longer useful.

Sonnie, JoAnn, and I went to Stanford last week to continue with the research project we started back in July 2005. We talked with her doctor, and he gave Sonnie her memory test. She didn't do very well.

She is at the stage where there isn't much the doctors can do for her.

Everything we can do; we can discuss over the phone. We will communicate by the phone and email every few months. Unless he wants specifically to see her, we won't need to make the trip to Stanford again.

Here are some comments on Sonnie's condition:

1) She is still a very beautiful lady.
2) Physically she is the same. Her weight is down to 100 pounds.
3) During the big fire down by our cabin she fell twice; both times she went head over heels.
   a. The first time I was clearing suckers from around the base of redwood trees, and she decided to help. She stepped off the side of the

trail and when I looked up, she was in the air. When she hit the ground, she was rolling and sliding. I was able to stop her slide just before she would have gone over the road bank to a straight fall of some eight to ten feet. Only a little blood, no other damage!

    b. The next fall came when I was working near one of our water tanks. Again, she wanted to help. And again, head over heels, only this time I was closer and stopped her slide right away. No blood.

4)   We were at a restaurant, and she was in the restroom doing her thing. When she came out the only thing holding up her pants was her belt. The fly of her pants was open exposing her underpants and her underpants were showing above her belt line. I came to her rescue! With her back to the wall and me on one knee in front of her, I undid her belt so I could button her pants and zip them up, plus push her underpants below her belt line. She had her hands down to hide everything that was happening. I said, "Sonnie you have to raise your hands so I can see what I'm doing." Her hands shot straight up over her head into the air. At that point I thought that I would probably get shot or arrested or something. Joni was here and we bought some pants that she can just pull up, but I'm still nervous about public restrooms.

5)   We were at the cabin, and I was working on putting in a double-pane window. I came inside to check

on how she was doing. She said that she was having trouble with her feet. I sat her in a chair to look at her feet. It turned out that instead of socks, she had put one of those maxi pads that people wear for protection in their underwear in one shoe and the pad wrapper in the other. I simply told her that I thought it might be better if we put on some white socks to match her shirt. She felt that would be a good idea, and all was well.

6) Sonnie used to brush her teeth two or three times a day. Now trying to brush her teeth is like pulling them.

7) I think one of the hardest things I will come up against is trying to figure out what she wants to say. I anticipate there will be a time when the only way I'll know that she needs to go to the bathroom is if her knees are together.

8) I'm trying to figure out a way to install small personal portable travel toilets in the car and pickup truck for emergencies. I don't want to buy a van or motor home because I know that we would only need it for a few months. Any ideas?

We may have another cliffhanger ahead of us, but we won't know that for a few more days. She had her mammography test the week before last and a second one last week followed by an ultrasound. Ah, the golden years are not that golden. After that experience, I spoke to the doctor, and we won't be doing that anymore.

We haven't gotten another dog yet and I don't know if we will. Sonnie asks me nearly every day if I fed the dog. I don't know what to do about another dog yet.

That is enough for today. We love you all.

- Just me, Steve

The Perfect Pet

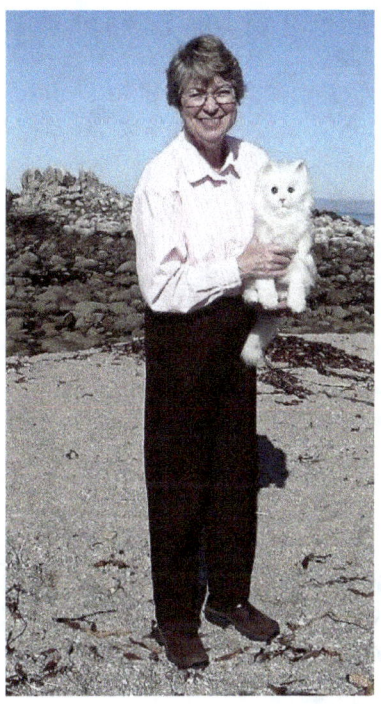

Sonnie and Poopsy at the beach
circa 2008

Shortly after Smoky died, Mom and Dad were in Walmart. Dad would take her through the toy aisle to see if anything caught her attention. She heard a cat meow. She looked up and held out her arms. Dad put a mechanical toy cat into her arms. She once again had the perfect pet.

I told Dad he might want to purchase two in case that one got broken or lost. She carried it everywhere. That cat even got buckled into the seatbelt with her.

She had a small collection of little stuffed animals she liked. They went everywhere with her including at the dinner table and to the beach.

Mom loved the beach. Dad took her there a couple of times a week. They would look for shells and play in the waves. One time, she almost went forward instead of backwards as the wave washed ashore. He caught her and pulled her back with only a little water on their feet. After that, he kept her back from the waves.

Mom kept a shoe box full of cards, Christmas cards, birthday cards, any cards. She would sit at the kitchen table and Dad would bring out her box of cards. She spent hours looking through her "mail" and attempting to write back. We still have several cards with her scribbles as she tried to write.

As the disease progressed, Mom slowly started to just want to be at home in Salinas where she was most comfortable. The mountains and cabin were Dad's happy place. She preferred to be in town.

When she wanted something, she wanted it NOW. She had lost the ability to be patient and to wait. If they were at their cabin, when she was ready to go back to Salinas, she would start walking down the road. Dad didn't have time to finish packing or even lock the door. If he turned his back, she was gone. Slowly, they went less and less to the cabin until they stopped going altogether.

- Joni

Email Update #8: November 21, 2008

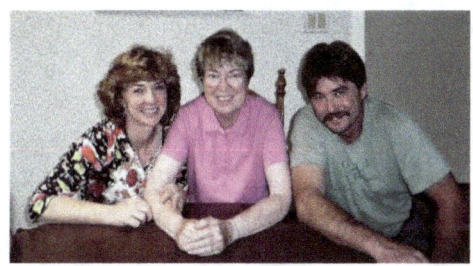

From left to right:
Joni, Sonnie and Jake
circa 2008

It's only been a little over two months since my last update, but a lot has happened.

Let me first thank everyone for the birthday cards that Sonnie received. It was overwhelming for her; she would laugh, cry, and a little bit of both at the same time. The cards that made noise or sang a tune would scare her at first and then she loved them. She received 29 cards, and we still look at them often.

Sonnie has trouble reading so I read whatever she wants. I can't get her interested in Zane Gray or Louis L'Amour; she likes Catherine Coulter and Nora Roberts. I never could understand women.

Thanks to many of you who sent me ideas for bathroom emergencies while traveling. I bought a light-weight plastic commode from Wal-Mart for under $20, and it holds all the extras we might need, like toilet paper, wet ones, even paper towels. I had more of a problem selecting the protective underwear. They have all these different brand names: Depends, Always, and Assurance. I finally decided that I could Always Depend on Assurance and went with Assurance.

Now I need to tell you about Sonnie's comfort kitty. It's a toy made by FurReal and looks like a real cat. We got it at Wal-Mart. Poopsy (Sonnie named it) will meow, blink her eyes, purr, knead with her paws and hiss if you grab her tail. We take Poopsy just about everywhere. The one problem with Poopsy is that she is kind-of awkward to carry around. I think that we may have solved that problem! Thanks to Prudy, I got in contact with Amie's Muttsy Mission for Alzheimer's [2] in Michigan and ordered a Muttsy for Sonnie. Well, I'll tell you all about Muttsy in my next update after I get him and see how Sonnie takes to him.

---

[2] Unfortunately, at the publishing of this book, this organization is no longer active.

Sonnie is into wandering now. She has wandered three times; all three times have been from our cabin. The first time she only got about a hundred yards; the second time she got close to a quarter ¼ mile and the last time she came close to a half mile. There aren't too many ways she can go, and she isn't into going uphill, but if she made a sharp right or left off the road in some places, it could be a long drop down the mountain. Bob and Julie gave me a tip on a GPS tracking watch that sounds good. First, I'm going to look into a device that the Monterey County Sheriffs have for finding people. I have the Chaperone option through my Verizon cell phone, but we don't get cell service at the cabin in the mountains.

After all the testing at the mammography center, Sonnie's lump is normal/benign.

I've spoken with our doctor at Stanford, and we decided to wean Sonnie off the Exelon medication to benefit her quality of life. The drug doesn't seem to be helping her much cognitively at this point anyway, and maybe I can get her weight up a little. Our doctor here in Salinas has taken her off the Wellbutrin and I have already seen her tremors subside. We'll go back to the doctor and see how she is doing one month from now and go from there.

Here are some examples on her condition:

1) I just can't believe with all that is going on in her head she can stay so beautiful. If you met us on the street or in a store you would think she was just fine.
2) Her weight is still 100 pounds.
3) I don't know if she was hiding from me or just sitting on the floor in the sun enjoying the warmth, but the other day she would not answer my call. When I found her, she was sitting on the floor at the end of the couch where I couldn't see her, close to the sliding glass door with her hands on her knees just looking out the glass door at whatever. I just sat on the floor next to her and we talked. I don't remember what about, we just talked.
4) What happens when you put lipstick on the lips of a beautiful woman – it enhances her beauty? When that same woman puts lipstick under and around her eyes, it seems to take something away, except maybe on Halloween.
5) We take our showers together when I wash her hair, about every three days. A couple weeks ago I was getting everything ready, setting the water temperature, etc. Well, she got in and one of us must have bumped the hot water control. She screamed, jumped out of the shower, ran in the bedroom, and locked the door. I shut everything down, got out and knocked on the door. She opened it and ran past me screaming "Who are you! What are you doing to me?" and headed for the

front door (naked). Fortunately, I had put double keyed locks on all the doors a couple of weeks before (thanks Judy for the suggestion!). It took a while to calm her down so I didn't try to wash her hair until the next day. No problem the next day; it was like nothing had happened. Can you picture Sonnie running down the street naked and me (naked) trying to catch her, with her hating me at that moment? That might have been too much excitement for the neighborhood that early in the morning.

6) This one I was going to leave out, but it is part of the Journey: the bathroom, more specifically the toilet. I don't know if it is the medication, my cooking, or her constitution, but Sonnie's stool is soft and sometimes leaves spots above the water line. Normally she doesn't remember to flush the toilet but on occasion she does, and twice now I have found her cleaning the spots in the toilet off with her bare hands and fingers. I don't kiss her fingertips as often as I did in the past to let her know that I love her; I kiss her forehead now! You must look on the bright side, though – our toilet bowls are spotless!

7) While I am not religious, I do take Sonnie to church every Sunday, and have for the last four years. She is a member of the Lutheran Church of the Good Shepherd. I go simply for her comfort and to point out where she is on the program. Communion is very important to her but over the last several

months she has been afraid to go forward and receive Communion. At first, I would ask one of the women members of the church if they would walk with her and each time they did and they were all great. About a month ago there was no one around us so I walked with her. Can you imagine the thoughts going through my mind – "Will lightning strike?" "Will the big quake hit?" Well, nothing happened! I just stood behind her, she received Communion and we returned to our seat. Where did the word pew come from anyway?

I will be sticking a lot closer to Sonnie over the next few months, or however long it takes for her emotion and anxiety levels to balance out. I would not feel comfortable leaving her with anyone right now. I'm still learning how to handle her catastrophic reactions. A rain shower to us is like a hurricane to her. JoAnn gave me a book "The 36-Hour Day" by Nancy L. Mace and Peter V. Rabins, and it is good. If you know of anyone caring for someone with dementia, tell them to get the book or get it for them.

Enough, enough. Everyone have a great Thanksgiving,

We love you all.

– Just me, Steve

Losing Best Friends

My grandmother used to say, "getting old is for the birds," and that "the golden years are not all that golden." Everyone dies eventually. The longer you live, the more friends you will lose, until one day you look around and so many of the people you love and grew up with are gone.

Losing his best friends was hard on Dad. I know he would have liked to have gone to Ben's Celebration of Life, but with Mom's condition deteriorating, it just wasn't in the cards.

- Joni

<u>Email Update #9: December 16, 2008</u>

This update is more for me than Sonnie.

It's been about a month since my last update.

This time I just need to talk, to talk about him, me, us, and them.

On the night of Wednesday, December 3rd, or maybe it was Thursday, Ben passed away in his bed at home. I don't know all the details, but I choose to believe that he passed away peacefully in his sleep. My guess is that it was a heart attack. Just over a year ago, his wife Lois passed away of complications from leukemia.

Ben was our best man when Sonnie and I were married coming up on 47 years. He was only 72 years old and that is young by today's standards. Ever since Lois died, Ben and I would talk on the phone at least once a week and sometimes more. We would talk about the weather, our kids, our grandkids, and our days in the fire service.

A couple months ago he was looking forward to going back to work for FEMA (Federal Emergency Management Agency) after his vacation to visit Gary (his son) and family in Hawaii. He called me when he got home, and I asked if he was ready for FEMA and if FEMA was ready for him. He said no, he didn't think he could give 100% and that traveling isn't what it used to be, so he thought he would pass, at least for a while. I called him on Monday, and we just talked for a few minutes because he had a doctor's appointment to get the results of some blood work. Now he's gone.

I didn't take the chance to go to his Celebration of Life in Redding. I couldn't leave Sonnie and she wouldn't have been able to make the trip. So, Sonnie and I went to where Lois is resting in Monterey. We left some flowers and visited awhile to support the end of their Journey. Ben will be placed next to Lois.

Ben's daughter Tami and her family kept him busy. When we would talk on the phone, he would tell me all about the football games, basketball games, track meets and whatever else was going on with the grandkids. He missed a game – that's how Tami and Tim, her husband, found him. Ben missed a game, and they went to his house. If medals could be given out to daughters and their families for watching over dads, Tami and her family would get the gold.

I'll think of Ben every day, as I do Lois, Ron, Juan, and many others. The sad thing is the names I just wrote are all younger than I am and had so much to live for...

Our Journey Continues:

Time sure goes by fast, but I was stumped a couple of weeks ago when Sonnie asked me, "What is time?" I tried to explain "time" several different ways until finally I decided I didn't even know what time was. I knew what time it was; I just didn't know how we got there! I know when it is time to eat, and I look forward to when it is time to go to sleep.

Sonnie asked questions on all kinds of topics, but I was never sure how she received my answers because she would go on to something else or just sit quiet right after she asked the question.

Cooking becomes more exciting every day. She wants to help, and I want her to help, but I think I'll give up on cooking rice (the 20-minute kind). She can take the lid off the pot within seconds from when I explain why she shouldn't. For now, I just keep testing it until it is soft enough not to break our teeth and drain the water off.

Sonnie's weight is 104 pounds, up from 100 and mine is 175 pounds, down from 180. Not bad for less than a month. It seems that I am having trouble with gravity, my shoulder and chest muscles have slipped and forced my stomach down to where I must bend over a little to see my belt buckle. I don't feel too bad though since Sonnie hasn't escaped the effects of gravity either.

About two weeks ago Sonnie was really depressed. I couldn't get her to stop crying. She finally got it across

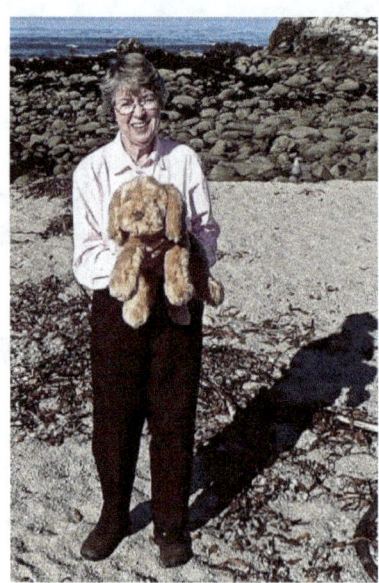

Sonnie and Muttsy at the beach
circa 2008

Sonnie's Journey

to me that she was so lonely that she thought she would go crazy. She wanted me to call the doctor or a counselor. I called my best friend at the Alzheimer's Association for help. She came through, like she always does, and suggested that I try taking her to the Adult Care Services Center managed by The Visiting Nurse Association. So far, so good. Sonnie's problem is that when she wants to go home, she wants to go home now, even if she doesn't know where home is. We'll see how it goes; they may just send her home!

She loves Muttsy, Poopsy and Pee-Wee. I told you about Poopsy in my last up-date but none of you know about Pee-Wee.

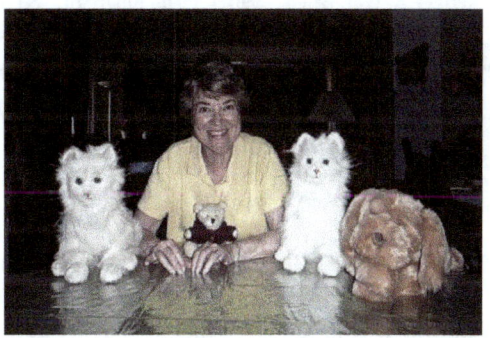

Poopsy, Sonnie, Pee-Wee, Susie, and Muttsy, Circa 2009

Pee-Wee is a little bear that Sonnie won playing bingo at the adult center last week and is now the third member of our in-home family. When I picked Sonnie up the day she won Pee-Wee she was sitting in a chair with her red jacket on holding the little bear in her arms like you would an infant. Now Pee-Wee is only about six inches long and I wish I had a picture of her sitting in that chair holding that little bear. It was something to see.

I almost forgot to tell you about Muttsy. Muttsy is perfect. He is a lap dog about two feet long, golden tan and is as soft and cuddly as anything I would ever want to hold (except for Sonnie of course).

But more important is Fran Maier. This woman is fantastic. In 2008 Fran maintained a website, muttsy.org[3], where she posted an article about "Amie's Mission," as well as all her accomplishments and her dreams for the future. She sent us a CD, "Music for Muttsy's" by Fran Maier, with our Muttsy. She has a beautiful voice. Sonnie and I played the CD at least a dozen times; I don't know how to say thanks to Fran and her organization for "remembering those who no longer can" (her words). Unfortunately, the organization and the website are no longer active.

It's important to me that you know that Sonnie is very easy to take care of most of the time. As we travel through this Journey you read about the traumatic times and the good times. We still have good times. We even dance now, in our family room, while listening to "Music for Muttsy".

---

[3] Unfortunately, this organization is no longer active

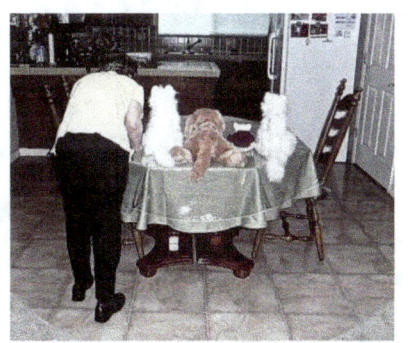

Sonnie chatting with friends,
a rear view, circa 2009

I'm going to leave you with "A Woman's Prayer" author unknown. Sonnie placed this prayer on our refrigerator door years ago, before Alzheimer's, in a spot where I would be sure to see it:

"A Woman's Prayer"

Dear Lord, I pray for:
Wisdom to understand my man.
Love to forgive him.
Patience for his moods.
Because Lord, if I pray for Strength,
I'll beat him to death.

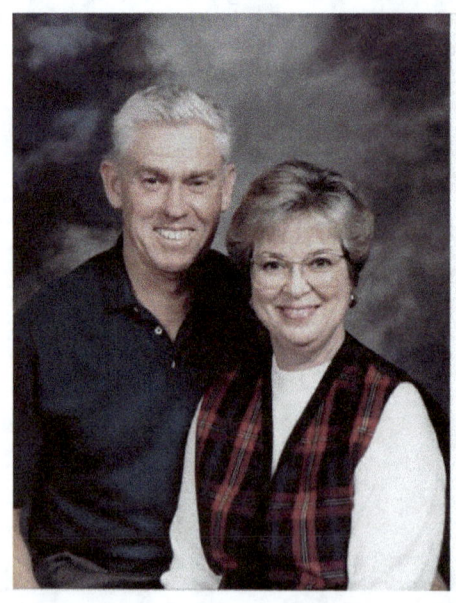

Sonnie's Journey

PS: Joni will be here in a few days, and maybe we can come up with a Christmas card showing at least some of our family. It may be late, but our thought and our hope is that all of you have the best Christmas that you can.

We love you all,

- Just me, Steve

How Important Is a Big Bathroom? VERY

The bathroom. One of those places you don't think about much, even though you need it multiple times each and every day. You use it for the toilet, shower, bath, washing your hands, brushing your teeth, fixing your hair, and getting ready to go somewhere.

Dad's right, we need to think about things differently as we get older, especially if we are caregivers.

At the top of the list of things to think about is the bathroom.

- Joni

<u>Blog entry</u>

If I were young and buying a house that I thought I might grow old in, or if I were older and looking for a home to live in for the rest of my life, I would buy a home with a big, big bathroom. This is a must!

Our bathroom is about 8 feet by 5 feet, and there isn't much room to move around.

Joni and her son Jake, then 16, came to visit just before Christmas. Jake helped me make some changes to our bathroom. We took the door off and replaced it with an accordion door. The regular door opened in and took up what seemed like half the room. If I were to build a bathroom today it would be at least 10 feet by 12 feet with all the trimmings and a drain in the middle of the floor. Grandkids grow up fast; Jake read the directions to install the door and even did most of the work. It felt good working with him; he is not a boy anymore but a young man, and a good one.

I bought a small computer chair that I could roll through the opening to enter the bathroom. Toward the end of her Journey, I would roll Sonnie into the bathroom so I could get her on the bench in the bathtub to wash her. I thought I was going to have to take out the toilet to move around enough just to make it safe to give her a bath and shower.

We were a little more than four years into our Journey and one morning I went in to get Sonnie up for breakfast. She looked up at me from the bed and said, "I'm going to die today". That was pretty heavy! I asked if she felt bad and she said "yes," and her eyes really looked sad. I sat down on the bed next to her and said, "Do you think that you could wait until this afternoon? We have a doctor's appointment this morning at 10:15." I got what I call "the Sonnie look" and she smiled and said "OK".

-Just me, Steve

Who Are You?

Dad always tried to keep on a happy face and for the most part was successful. I know he did what he could to insulate me from the worst of what he was experiencing as Mom's caregiver. I know I got the edited version.

Mom and Dad were usually in bed asleep by 8:00 pm. So, when the phone rang after 8 and it was Dad, I knew there was a big problem.

Slowly losing my mother and watch her get replaced by a shell was tough. Answering the phone to hear my Dad say, "Talk to your mother, she doesn't know who I am," was the toughest.

- Joni

Email Update #10: January 15, 2009

When I first started out writing "Sonnie Updates" it was just once a year, then twice a year, and now it seems like one every few months. What I do is write notes on a pad next to my computer, and when I get about what I think is two pages worth I sit down and put something on the computer.

The other day I had a very interesting, good, and challenging day. Picture, if you will, a perfect day for

January. The temperature was around 72 degrees, no wind, or clouds, just a nice, beautiful day.

Sonnie and I woke up around six thirty in the morning or so and just stayed in bed and talked until about eight. We decided to go and stay overnight at our cabin. On the way there we would stop and have lunch on the beach south of Carmel.

Our first stop was at Home Depot to buy a couple of deadbolt locks (double keyed) to install at the cabin to help prevent Sonnie from wandering. The next stop was at the grocery store to buy whatever we hadn't brought from home. The third stop was to pick up lunch. Lunch consisted of a foot-long Subway sandwich cut into four pieces. The last stop was the beach for a picnic lunch.

The beach was great. The water was a clear light jade green, the ocean was calm, and the sand was warm. We ate part of our sandwich and talked. I would tell her about past events and places we've seen. She would say – "Yes, Steve and I have done that too." Or "We've done that too." Or "My husband and I have done that too." We stayed at the beach for about an hour then drove on and stopped at a place where we could walk along and look down at the ocean. We talked, of course, and again Sonnie would answer as before. "Yes, Steve and I have done that too." Or "We've done that too." Or "My husband and I have done that too."

Once we arrived at the cabin, we got the groceries, and everything put away in its place. I was going to drill the holes for the deadbolts and install them, but we had a leak in our water line just outside the cabin, so first things first I fixed the water line, then installed the deadbolts. After that, I puttered around for the rest of the afternoon. When we finished dinner, I was going to have a small fire in our fire pit on the patio so we could sit and watch the moon rise over the mountains, but the wind was a little stronger than I liked, so we sat on our swing under the apple tree instead. It was a good day, and a nice evening.

Then it got challenging. It must have been around eight o'clock when I suggested that we brush our teeth and get ready for bed. Normally we go to bed around eight and talk until nine or ten before falling asleep.

Sonnie said she couldn't go to bed; she would have to wait for her husband. I tried to explain that I was Steve, her husband, and even showed her my driver's license. I didn't have any pictures that would help. I told her that I was her husband and that we had two children. I told her we had a son and a daughter. That got her attention. I asked her if she wanted to talk to her daughter. She said "Yes!" so I called Joni for help.

Joni talked to her mother. She told her that the man standing in front of her was her husband. She said "I'm your daughter and that's my dad. He's your husband." Joni even had her looking at her wedding rings to see if they would ring a bell. When they finished talking, I thought the problem was solved. Apparently not as a few minutes later, I could tell by her eyes, she still wasn't sure if I was her husband or her friend. The only thing left to do was to pack up, go home and hope for the best.

It must have been around ten-thirty when we got home. It seemed like another world to Sonnie. It took me at least ten minutes to convince her that this was our home. I thought I was going to have to sleep on the daybed in the computer room for a while, but it all worked out. I still don't know if she knew I was her husband or if sleeping with a friend was better than sleeping alone.

The next morning it was as if nothing had happened.

At this point in our Journey, the Adult Day Care Services stopped working out. The last three times I took her, I could tell that she wasn't happy. One time when we arrived, as soon as she looked in the door, she was ready to go home.

Now we will go to Plan B. I just need to come up with a Plan B first.

If anyone has an idea as to how Sonnie could still have some independence and not be so lonely, let me know. Neither Sonnie nor I want to ask people to stop by for short visits and it is hard for me to ask if we can stop by and visit other people for a few minutes. Groups aren't her bag. It is not unusual for friends and neighbors to stay away—they just don't know what to say or talk about. Plus, Sonnie can't put a full sentence together. Our circle is getting smaller and smaller.

- Just me, Steve

Yoooou Whoooo, Is Anyone Here?

Dad always tried to keep Mom engaged and involved. If I called, even though Mom couldn't carry-on or follow a conversation, he would hand her the phone. I would chat for a while, until Dad would come back on the line as Mom would set down the phone, hand it back or walk away. Her mind had lost the thread and moved on to something else. There was very little that would hold her attention.

While she may not know who I was if you told her about me, there is no doubt in my mind, or Dad's, that she always knew my voice, to the very end. So, I kept calling and talking, even if it was to myself.

- Joni

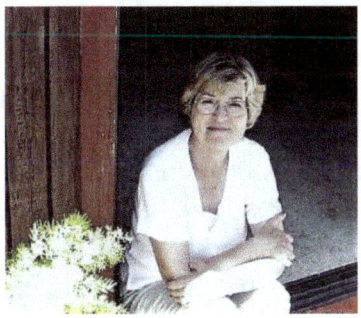

Sonnie circa 2008

Blog entry

Sonnie whistles. She didn't whistle before, but now she does. She is pretty good at it, too. I don't think I have ever heard her whistle before.

The first time was when she was looking for me. I would hear a couple of whistles followed by a "Yoooou Whoooo, is anyone here?" Then she would whistle a tune. Not bad.

I met a lady that had taken care of her mother with Alzheimer's, and she gave me a good analogy for Alzheimer's. "Think of Alzheimer's as a large circle and as that circle spirals inward, very slowly, it will come to an end with nothing but a dot in the center." I didn't know at the time where Sonnie was in our Journey as it spirals to the center, but I had to expect the unexpected. I just wasn't sure when to expect it.

One evening Joni called to say hi and give us a run down on our grandkids. After she and I talked a while, I went in the kitchen to give Sonnie the phone. Sonnie's hands were wet from helping with the dishes, so I handed her a hand towel and told her that Joni wanted to talk to her. Sonnie took the towel, held it up to her ear and said, "Hi Joni." She said it several times before I could trade the phone for the towel. She did that another time with a bar of soap.

- Just me, Steve

I'm Sick, Aren't I?

I grew up in what I call a balanced religious environment. Mom was Catholic until her parents died, then she switched to Lutheran. I think of Lutherans as being Catholic without all the guilt. Either way, church was an important part of her life. Mom sang in the choir and had a beautiful voice.

Dad was not raised with a religion. In fact, Grandma claimed she was an atheist. He only appeared in church for weddings and funerals.

When Mom stopped driving, Dad started taking her to church because it was important to her. He took her every Sunday as long as they were able. And when they were no longer able to attend church, he arranged for the pastor or lay person to stop at the house to say a few prayers with her and give her communion.

Dad always made sure that things important to Mom, or that made her happy, happened.

- Joni

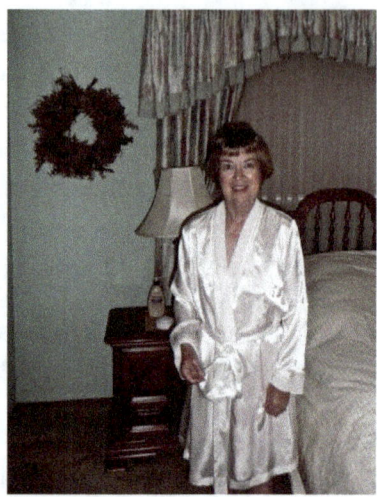

Sonnie circa 2008

One morning when I went to the bedroom to get Sonnie up for breakfast she asked, or rather told me, "I'm sick, aren't I."

I didn't know if she meant sick to her stomach or sick with Alzheimer's or sick of me!

Then she said something like, am I going to die, or I want to die, something in the line of dying anyway. There were a few months that she mentioned death or dying several times.

She would talk about when "we" get to heaven. Not being religious, I would try to put a little humor in my answers and say things like "You say 'we', are you going to have a baby?" or "Sonnie, I've been a Fireman all my life. I may have one more challenge facing me at the Gates of Hell." But sometimes even humor doesn't help.

Most of the time when I brought God into the picture, things would become a little clearer for her and then we could move on to her next moment.

- Just me, Steve

The Digital Picture Frame

Mom's ability to communicate was slowly deteriorating. She could no longer form words. You could see, in her eyes, how frustrated she would get. But that too would quickly fade, and she would simply give up.

I was going through a phase where I didn't want to look old, so I was trying out a new eye cream at night. I had gotten ready for bed and had applied my eye cream. It made the skin around my eyes red.

Mom was already tucked into bed. I went in to tell her goodnight and give her a kiss. When I bent down to give her a kiss, she looked at me with concern in her eyes. Then touched my face near my eyes. I said, "Oh that, I'm using a new eye cream. I don't mind getting old, but I do mind getting ugly." She understood and smiled. It was one of the last times I saw her smile.

- Joni

Email Update #11: April 07, 2009

It's been about four years and six months since Sonnie was diagnosed.

The Journey is moving right along. My notes pile up here by the computer, but my time to write is limited. Right now Sonnie is still in bed asleep and my guess is that in order for me to keep my "Support Group" up-to-date, I'll do my writing at night or early in the morning.

She needs my full attention now. She will wander through the house always looking for something to do, or at least move.

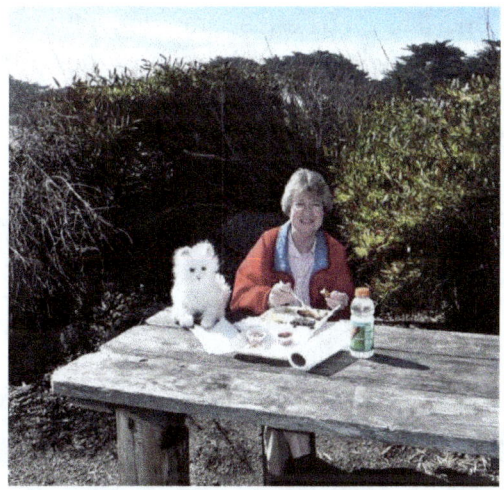

Sonnie circa 2008

I knew something was wrong way back in January of 2003 when she couldn't find where the pot holders were kept. I might think that I have Alzheimer's now, except I know where the pot holders are supposed to be, I just can't find where she put them!

I told you about the time that she almost brushed her teeth with Desitin. I didn't catch her in time to prevent her from moisturizing her teeth with Aveeno. No harm done.

I'm glad that our stove has a lock; At different times I found the burners left on. Fortunately neither time was for very long. Now I make it a point to lock the surface burners.

We go out to dinner once or twice a month with our best friends Joe and JoAnn. The last time we went out, on the way home Sonnie was saying how nice "those people" were and that she would like to go out to dinner again with them sometime.

You know Spray and Wash, that stuff you spray on your clothes when they get stained or extra dirty? I buy it by the gallon. I've always been a little messy, and now Sonnie has a habit of trying to match the front of her shirt to look like mine. Usually it is when we are sitting on the couch watching TV and I give her a dish of ice cream with chocolate syrup on top.

A MUST HAVE when you are caring for someone with dementia is a Digital Picture Frame! Joni gave us one. It was ready to go with lots of pictures loaded onto the memory card. We keep it by the computer. Jake gave us one (also ready to go) that we keep by the couch in the family room. I don't remember how many pictures they hold, but they are set up as slide shows and we spend a lot of time watching things from our past. Jake's wife, Cheryl, scanned pictures taken years ago from albums when Sonnie was a baby, and even some of her old boyfriends, and they are all on this little microchip. What will they think of next?

Sonnie's communication skills are slowly falling by the wayside. We had a floral design on our bedsheets. The design was all the same color (a light blue) and spread evenly throughout the sheets. Several times she took me in and showed me the flowers, thinking that something was wrong. We put on plain white sheets, and she was happy and probably even slept better.

One night, shortly after midnight, she got up to go to the bathroom. She passed up a perfectly good bathroom, complete with a nightlight, and ended up in the dining room sitting on a dining room chair. I always call to her after a while to ask if everything is OK. This time her voice seemed too far away so I got up and found her just sitting there very confused. Did you know that a bladder holds enough fluid to go through a nightgown, bathrobe, and chair cushion, and still get some on the floor? I gently got her back to the bathroom, cleaned her up with a washcloth and got her back to bed. Then I went back and got the dining room cleaned up and ready for breakfast.

Two days later I was checking my email about midafternoon when she came in and wanted to "show me the water." "Water" has many meanings for Sonnie. I got up and followed her towards the bedroom but we stopped at the clothes hamper just outside the bathroom door. We had just completed the washing that morning so when she opened the hamper, I was surprised to see a pair of underpants in the bottom of the hamper and on the underpants she had left a deposit and around her deposit was the water she wanted to show me. It would seem to me to be very uncomfortable to sit on a hamper and have a bowel movement, but it can be done.

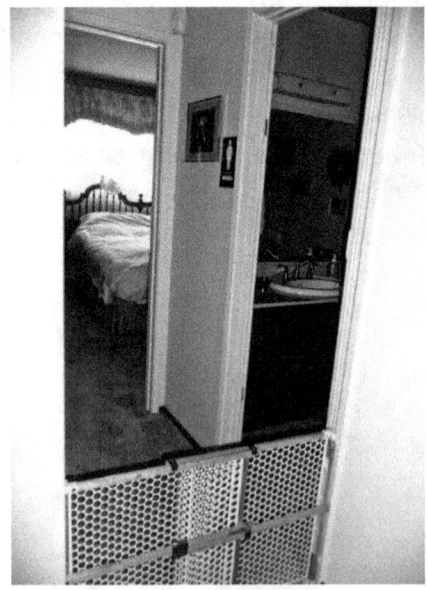

Hallway gate

I started making it a point to have her go to the restroom about every three hours. I was talking to Dorothy, my sister, and she suggested that I get one of those fences they use for children and put it across the hall to guide her towards the bathroom. It worked perfectly. The night light from the bathroom lights it up good enough to where she won't trip over the fence in the dark—another good idea!

I'm going to get one of those potty chairs to put by the bed so she can see it from any part of the hallway. We had one when we were caring for Dad and Mom; I'll have to check and see if we still have it. We had what they call a "hospital bed" at one time. It will come in handy somewhere down the road. I'll have to check with Jake to see if we still have that, too. As you can tell, my memory is fading with age.

If you were to watch Sonnie eat you would think that she had Parkinson's disease. Her tremors are getting worse. At night her whole body twitches every few minutes. I don't know how she sleeps as good as she does. I know she sleeps a lot better than I do. I get between two and six hours of sleep a night. I rest a lot during the day!

A few days ago Sonnie fell while coming down the steps at Joe and JoAnn's. She landed pretty hard on her right side. We checked her out good before we left, and she was able to walk ok. When we got home I had her take off her clothes and found that her right hip and forearm were starting to bruise. Now she has two black and blue marks. The good thing is—she doesn't remember falling. I normally help her down steps and curbs, but not that day. I let myself get distracted.

I've gone over my two page limit, so I'll cut my notes off here and give everyone a break.

- Just me, Steve

I Need to Go Home NOW

At this point, Mom had completely lost her ability to communicate.

Occasionally she would say something that we could figure out, but for the most part she was silent.

I do believe that she always knew Dad, my brother and I were somehow important to her. She may not always have known who we were and why we were important, but she knew we were somehow special. The day before she died, I walked into the room and said, "Hi Mommy," and her head snapped up. Maybe it was coincidental or maybe I just startled her; we'll never know. I choose to believe, and Dad agrees, that while she may not have known my face, she always knew my voice.

- Joni

Email Update #12: May 6, 2009

My notes keep adding up. I know it has only been one month since my last update, but I'll never catch up if I don't keep up.

Sonnie's life (our life) can be compared to that of a prisoner. Our exercise amounts to walking around the neighborhood for thirty minutes, maybe an hour on a good day.

Her mind must be trying to go a mile a minute just wanting to escape to something that is familiar, something that she can cling to. It must be frustrating, particularly now that it's difficult for her to communicate even a simple sentence.

All these years, whenever I cooked, I've tried to have the meat, potatoes, salad, and vegetable prepared and ready to put on the table at the same time. Now, sometimes that's good and sometimes not so good. I might be better off to just have one dish at a time for her to eat. If they are all on her plate, she might mix them together like stir fry or place one item on her napkin and another in her glass of water. We always wash the lettuce before we put it in the salad. Sonnie likes to help make the salad, but she wants to wash the lettuce after the salad is made and that takes something away from the delivery.

A couple weeks ago we had another first—she would not use her utensils and ate her dinner with her hands. That wasn't too bad with the chicken and broccoli, but the salad and potatoes were a little tough to handle.

JoAnn was in the hospital for about five days a few weeks ago, and Sonnie and I went to see her every day. When we got to the hospital, I put hand sanitizer on my hands and then put a little in the palm of Sonnie's hand. Right away her hand went up to her mouth and I said, "NO, no, no don't eat it!" but she did get a little in her mouth before I could stop her. I had to find a water

Sonnie's Journey

fountain to rinse her mouth out. The funny thing was that when we got to JoAnn's room, I was telling her and Joe about our experience and I demonstrated what happened by putting a little squirt of hand sanitizer in Sonnie's hand. She did it again! This time I was able to catch her hand before it got to her mouth.

We did have another incident where there was a wet area on the carpet at the end of our bed. I found it with my bare feet while heading for the bathroom one evening. That was the feel test. I got down on my hands and knees and gave it the smell test with no results. No, I didn't give it the taste test. I soaked up what I could with old rags and paper towels. It's still a mystery.

I found that while driving, or at home for that matter, Christmas music and music that is sung by a choir is more soothing for her than other types of music. So, it's Christmas here year-round.

We were brushing our teeth before going to bed and she was looking at my stomach kind of funny. When we had finished with our teeth, she patted my stomach and asked if I was pregnant. And she meant it! I guess now I'll have to beware of stretch marks.

Sonnie is getting more and more afraid of going to church. She doesn't read anymore and it's hard to follow the program. There is a nice lady that takes her up for communion, but she is ready to panic when the usher gets close to our row. About a month ago she came back to her seat from communion, sat down, opened her hand, and gave me the wafer that the pastor had handed her.

"I need to go home now." She says that a lot and it doesn't necessarily mean to go to our house. I think she wants to do something else, to change the situation she's in and be in a more comfortable atmosphere. The biggest problem I have now is understanding what she is trying to communicate.

I'm registered and hope to go to a conference on "The Changing Face of Dementia." Sonnie's doctor from Stanford is going to be one of the keynote speakers and will speak about the diagnosis and treatment of Alzheimer's disease. Sonnie and I are very lucky to have excellent doctors.

Take care and if you hear of or think of anything about Alzheimer's and caregiving, let me know.

- Just me, Steve

The Last 6 Months

The last 6 months were bad.

Not even Dad, with his optimistic and cheerful outlook, could frame it any other way. No one should have to go through what Mom endured. She wouldn't have wanted to live like that, but with Alzheimer's, by the time you get there it's too late for you to choose a different path.

I was doing what I could from Phoenix. I was increasing my visits to every 2 months and preparing to go to every month so I could help Dad. With my job, I was fortunate enough to be able to work remotely.

My Mom was gone. I had lost my mother years ago. Dad was taking care of the shell that used to be my mother and killing himself in the process.

He insisted he was ok. I strongly suspected he wasn't telling me how bad it really was.

I was worried about Dad.

- Joni

Email Update #13: June 14, 2009

Sonnie and I both have Long Term Care Insurance and we have opened a claim in her name. Not so much because we need it at this point, but to make it easier on the kids if something happens to me. No, I'm not sick or anything like that—I just like to be prepared. Plus, there is a ninety-day elimination period on the policy.

It was neat the way all this happened. The insurance company called me to see if I would like an agent to come by and go over our policies with us. I told the young lady that would be a good idea because my wife has Alzheimer's. There was a pause… then she replied how sorry she was and asked me to wait a few minutes while she looked at the policy. She asked me a few questions, told me that this person and that person would be contacting me and bingo—we're set to go. We have our own Privileged Care Coordinator to work with us on the Alzheimer's Journey (or at least until the money runs out). Oh, the Golden Years!

I'm starting to see more and more physical movement problems with Sonnie. While we are walking, she often holds her right arm like she is getting ready to draw a six-shooter while the left arm swings merrily along. Getting in and out of the car has been something to watch now for some time—not just her movements but explaining the seat belt and where her arms need to be or not be. There is no sign of a stroke; I think it is just part of the disease.

I told you in the last update that I was going to get a potty chair and put it in the bedroom where she could see it from the hallway. I did. I went to the Goodwill Store and got one for twelve dollars. It looked like new, so we brought it home, sterilized it, and a few days later, it worked! She used the potty chair instead of something else.

We had popcorn a while back and she lost a filling from a back tooth. It didn't hurt her, but I could see by her actions that there was a problem). I was a little nervous at the dentist office because she's not into needles or pain, but it all worked out well, and now she is ready for more popcorn.

Going to church is just about a thing of the past. I get her up and ready every Sunday, but I know Communion scares her. She just can't remember what is expected of her. About three Sundays ago the lady that usually walks with her to Communion wasn't there, so I walked with her and stood behind her while she received Communion. The Pastor placed the wafer in her hand and went on to the next person. Sonnie held the wafer in her hand while the assistant came up to hand Sonnic the thimble of wine. She took the thimble as I kneeled and told her she needed to eat the wafer and drink the wine. By that time the girl came by with the container to pick up the empty thimble, so Sonnie reached over with her left hand to take an empty thimble from the container while her right hand was leaning to the right about to spill the wine in her full thimble on the carpet. I was reaching for the thimble in her right hand while explaining why she doesn't need an empty thimble and thinking — God, why? Here at your table, and me already waiting for an earthquake, lightning, or some other disaster to occur? We'll keep trying, but every time I ask her, she says "No, I don't feel like going right now."

Potpourri –You know the stuff that smells and is a combination of leaves, flower petals, and God knows what else. I found a package of some that Sonnie had stored in her China Cabinet. I thought it would be nice to put some in a small pot in our bedroom—wrong! Not more than a day or two later she was walking around the house with this red stuff in her mouth. I had no idea what it was, and to get something out of Sonnie's mouth once it's in there is NOT an easy job. But I did, and it was a red flower from the Potpourri. So much for another good idea.

Rock salt, too: I was adding salt pellets to our water softener and Sonnie was folding up the plastic sacks to be recycled. I must have missed a pellet, because there was Sonnie standing there having the time of her life sucking on this chuck of salt. She didn't want to give up her salt pellet, either.

We were at Joe and JoAnn's last week and we had some cake while we were there. When we were getting ready to start for home, everyone was standing around saying our goodbyes when Sonnie reached up her sleeve and wanted to know what to do with "this." Well, "this" was a fork we were missing after the cake was cut. Sonnie had slipped it under her Medic Alert bracelet, I guess to keep it in a safe place. I don't think she would begin to know how to steal something. Anyway, JoAnn got her fork back, the cake was good and the company better.

Occasionally, I'll take Sonnie to the Adult Day Care Center. She hates it but sometimes I just need the break or to get a few things done around the house.

Sonnie also hates when I'm in the computer room. One day, I was in the computer room doing the bills or something and it got quiet. If there is one thing I have learned as a caregiver, it's that if it gets quiet, you better get up and check. This time we didn't have a disaster, but it was very sad. When I got to the door of the room, I could see her in the mirror in the hall. She was sitting on the floor with knees drawn to her chest, just looking at the floor. So I went down the hall and simply sat across from her with my back to the mirror. She needs someone with her almost every minute; being close in the next room isn't good enough. So be it.

I took Sonnie for a drive over to Carmel a couple of weeks ago to the house where we were introduced.

The picture with the sign "Promises Kept" is where we met over dinner.

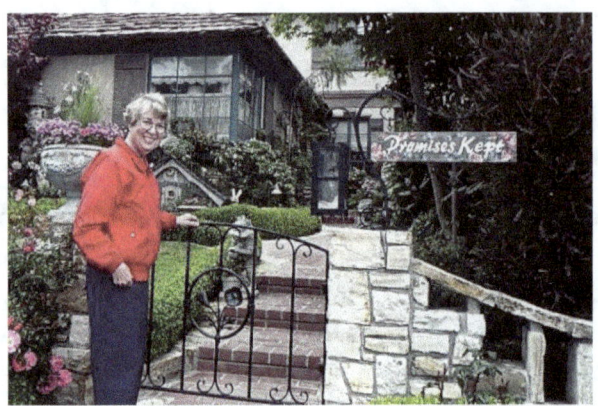

Carmel cottage Sonnie rented in 1962, circa 2009

The other picture is the cottage, behind the main house, where Sonnie was living. Behind the door to the cottage is where Sonnie and I first kissed. That's almost 48 years ago.

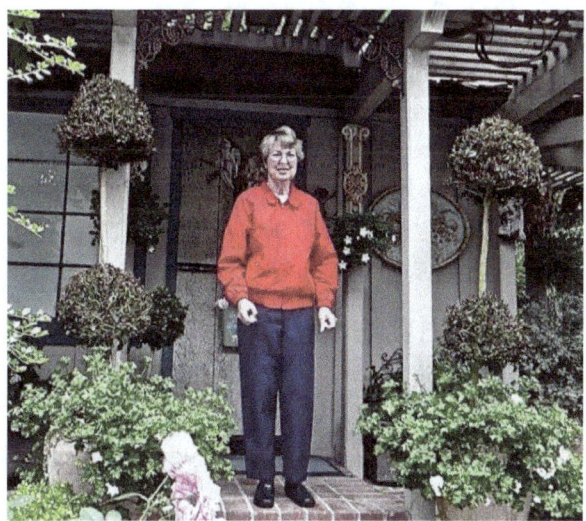

Carmel cottage Sonnie rented in 1962, circa 2009

The people that own the house now were very nice and allowed us to take these pictures.

I watched a special called "The Alzheimer's Project. It was good. There was one doctor that was a little more optimistic than I am. He seemed to suggest that a cure is just around the corner. All the stuff I read suggests if it's around the corner, it's a very far away corner.

- Just me, Steve

It's Been 5 Years

Everyone I know that has had a loved one go through Alzheimer's says the "angry phase" is terrible.

The summer of 2009 was extremely hard on Dad. He didn't say much about Mom's behavior. I found out the way everyone else did: through his updates.

I knew Mom could cuss like a sailor. Dad didn't see it as much as my brother and I did because he was off at work. Even though she couldn't put together a sentence, the colorful language she learned from her father came out loud and clear during this phase.

- Joni

Email Update #14: July 15, 2009

In two months, it will be five years since Sonnie was diagnosed with Alzheimer's. This last month has been the toughest so far. She has no patience at all, for anything. When we are stopped at a signal light, she wants me to "go, go—go—go!" I don't think she can distinguish between red and green, let alone amber. In a restaurant she wants to get up and leave before the food arrives. If she wants to go home (even if we are at home) it's right now; she gets her jacket and heads for a door. It may be a closet door, but it is a door.

I think the lack of patience has allowed anger to take over her normal personality. Since my last writing Sonnie has a "catastrophic reaction" (Alzheimer's talk) almost every day, and sometimes two or three. One day she wanted me out of the house and pushed me toward the door. Another time she hit me with a towel to keep me away. There was one afternoon I had to call Pat (my guardian angel) at the Alzheimer's Association for help. She came through, like she always does. She said to call a friend to come over and remove myself from the situation. My next call was to Rita to stop by and stand between us. I waited outside hiding behind the pickup. It took about five minutes and Rita had her purring like a kitten. It's good to have friends!

The reactions that Sonnie has now differ from earlier reactions in the way they start. Now it's like flipping a switch from off to on. Before they would take time to build up and I could adjust and make things a little more comfortable. Today I reach for a ½ pill of Xanax and hope for the best. I win a few and I lose a few. Fortunately, I took the "Savvy Caregiver Training Program" by the Alzheimer's Association and learned "don't argue, you can't win." Anyway, I'm starting to get a handle on how to deal with these catastrophic reactions and at least take off some of the pressure. I can see where the book titled "The 36 Hour Day" came from. My days are probably at the 30-hour mark and gaining.

Sonnie has taken up swearing. In all our years together, I have heard very few cuss words cross her lips. Most of those were spoken when she was sewing or hurt herself. She is (or was) one of those people that wouldn't say S--T even if she had a handful. She had four sisters and one brother so there must have been an opportunity to pick up one or two words along the way.

Another first – Sonnie forgot how to eat her breakfast. A couple of weeks ago I gave her oatmeal with raisins. She just stirred it with her spoon. I tried to show her what to do with the spoon and that didn't work. I finally fed her breakfast.

Sonnie does not understand what a lot of words mean. Some examples: Table, as in "set the table." She will walk right by the table every time. Sink, like "take this to the kitchen sink." She will head for the bedroom most of the time. Marriage, like man and wife. Maybe occasionally she seems to understand. Restroom—"Do you have to go?" Probably nine out of ten times I will have to show her where the toilet is located (not just the bathroom but the toilet). Just asking her if she needs to go to the bathroom doesn't get the job done anymore. Now I just take her every few hours and sometimes she goes and sometimes she doesn't.

Last week when we were washing our clothes, I had a close call. We use a liquid detergent (Gain) that is green in color. I had measured out the amount that we use in the clear cup provided and handed it to Sonnie so she could pour it in the machine. She held the cup for a few seconds and as I was turning away, I saw her out of the corner of my eye raising the cup to her lips. HARMFUL IF SWALLOWED! I stopped her just in time.

Susan sent me a nice email and suggested that Sonnie might like to tour the local animal shelters and visit the animals. So, I did, and she did. The only downside was the noise. As soon as I opened the door to the dog runs all barking broke loose and her hands went right to her ears. It just took a few minutes for her fear to subside and for her to enjoy most of the animals. Finding ways to entertain Sonnie is hard to do especially now that her fear level is so high. If you have any ideas, send them to me; a couple of them have to work.

Day care only lasted nine trips. It just isn't her bag. With the behavioral changes she is going through right now, I need to learn how to cope with these problems first before I hire or ask someone to stand in for me for any length of time. I know that I can call Pat at the Alzheimer's Association and she will help me when she can. JoAnn and Joe have been helping from day one. Rita and Jerry are calling, and we have been getting together these past few weeks. Plus, I have a list of people on "Sonnie's Care Plan" that would come if I needed them. I'm covered; I just want to do what I can first. I don't feel stressed but there are times I feel inadequate.

The morning after I sent the last "Sonnie Update," when I was getting Sonnie dressed, I noticed that she needed to blow her nose. I got her a Kleenex and told her, "Sonnie, you would look a lot prettier if you would blow your nose." Well, she held the Kleenex in her hand and just looked at me. I said "blow," and she did. She puckered up her mouth and blew out from her mouth. I said, "No, blow your nose" and she did. She puckered up her mouth, stuck out her tongue, pointed it toward her nose and blew from her mouth again. I finally held the Kleenex to her nose, and she got the idea.

Joni sent us another white kitty by FurReal in case Poopsy was to bite the dust. Sonnie liked it so much that it sits right next to Poopsy, Muttsy and Pee-Wee on the table. We named this one Susie after her sister to keep the "E's" going – Poopsy, Muttsy, Pee-Wee and now Susie. It goes with Sonnie and Stevie (my sister is the only one that still calls me Stevie).

I get Sonnie up and ready for church every Sunday. The last two Sundays that we did go we left when Communion started. One Sunday, we made it to the parking lot and last Sunday we did a drive-by. I'll try a few more times but I think God will have to take her as she is when the time comes.

It seems like the kitchen and the bathroom are where all the action happens. Three or four days ago she had been in the bathroom a little longer than normal, so I called and asked if everything was Ok. She said she didn't think so—I went in, and she was trying to pull her outer pants up with no luck. After a quick inspection I found a new bar of soap that she had wrapped with toilet paper and placed in her underpants preventing her from pulling her pants up. Sonnie has always liked that clean feeling!

- Just me, Steve

The Spiral Accelerates

August continued to be a tough month for Dad.

Mom's language wasn't the issue, the real problem was the violent behavior. I assume it's the frustration and brain chemistry changes that cause the "angry phase." However it happens, my understanding is that most Alzheimer's patients go through it. She was lashing out not just verbally but physically.

Dad finally found a medication that took the edge off her anger. He had to keep her on medication to control her temper. It lasted a few months and then, like everything else, time moved on, and he was able to wean her off the medication.

I only wish he had found the medication for her anger a couple of months earlier.

- Joni

Email Update #15: September 1, 2009

Where do you start—from today, and go back to July when I ended the last update, or follow my notes? The Journey lately has been like a car about to run out of gas; it will jerk and then run smooth for a while then jerk again and maybe run rough for a short distance. Right now, Sonnie is asleep on our bed. It's just after noon and she will sleep anywhere from fifteen minutes to an hour.

I go to a support group the first Wednesday of each month. Some of the caregivers say, "you have to learn how to lie." I can't seem to bring myself to lie to her yet but I'm getting pretty good at skirting the truth.

Here are some tips.

Sonnie used to dry her hair with the hair dryer. I was afraid she would use it with the water running in the sink for whatever reason, so I cut a piece of cardboard to set over the sink with the words "DO NOT TURN ON THE WATER" written with a marking pen. In hindsight it might have been better to just turn off the water under the sink. I haven't used the piece of cardboard in over a year. It was one of those short-term needs. Alzheimer's is the only long-term commitment.

Another thing I have been doing lately is pulling about two squares of toilet paper allowing them to hang from the roll. That way she is not looking at just a round roll of toilet paper.

Twice now Sonnie has unknowingly (I think) locked me out of the house. Last week I put an outdoor mini-key safe on the porch wall. I even put a key in the safe! Now I just must remember how to open it.

Not too long-ago Sonnie found another way to use lipstick—on her teeth!

She goes to bed sometimes as early as 7:30 pm. As she's laying down, just before her head reaches the pillow, she just drops the last six inches. She still sleeps pretty well most of the night and that's a help. She does have night sweats every few nights that soak the bed. These sweats are probably from a new medicine that we are trying, and hopefully will go away. I can't seem to find the right kind of waterproof pad that I want. Most of the ones on the market are 27" x 36". I want something about the size of a twin mattress cover so I can move her to a dry area to make it through the night. Right now, I am using a waterproof paint drop cloth. It's not really cloth but a soft paper on one side and plastic on the other. Then I put a flat twin mattress cover on top and that works.

In my last update I was telling you about Sonnie's "catastrophic reactions" and what a tough month it had been. Towards the end of July, we saw her doctor and I explained all that was happening. Now we are trying a very low dose (0.5MG) of an antipsychotic agent.

Two things happened; her anger has significantly reduced and her morning sickness that has been going on for two or three years is gone! The only obvious side effects are fatigue and night sweats. She gets tired easy. I have her take a nap just after lunch almost every day. She still goes to bed early and usually sleeps well. She seems to sleep on her back most of the night where before she liked to sleep on her right side.

Day care didn't work so I went to plan "B". Jean, a great lady that lives across the street, lost her mother last month. She had been caring for her mother and care giving for others over the years. She and I decided that she could help me, and she would be just across the street. She was going to start by coming over for about three hours twice a week.

Her first day was August 27th, from 1:00 to 4:00. I got the oil changed in the car and made three or four other stops and got home at four o'clock sharp. Poor Jean, the first two and a half hours went fine or at least OK. The last half hour was pure hell for Jean and Sonnie (I was doing great). Sonnie had a "catastrophic reaction" and it was a big one. When I walked in the door Jean was standing there and it wasn't long before Sonnie came in the room cussing, gesturing, and pushing Jean to get her out of the house. It wasn't a pretty sight. After Jean left, I must have filled the role that Rita did for me when Sonnie would get angry with me. I'm working on Plan "C" with JoAnn.

We went to JC Penny's the other day to look for a new comforter. The department we wanted was upstairs. We went up the escalator and looked around, didn't find anything we wanted and started to come back down. Sonnie would not get on the escalator. She would put her foot out like she wanted to, but she couldn't do it. Thankfully, we made it down in the elevator, instead.

Salinas had its annual air show not too long ago and we had our own private show here at the house. Every time the Blue Angels flew over, Sonnie's hands would go to her ears, and she would look for somewhere to hide. I found that it worked best to take her outside and point at the planes before they flew over. Any noise can make her jump. The show lasted four days.

Sonnie doesn't really walk anymore, she shuffles. We still go to the stores together but only one store at a time. We will come back home and rest between stores. It probably won't be too long before I'll have to go back to planning our shopping for a week at a time. Right now, I don't care if I only need one item. I'll save whatever it is I need until she needs to get out of the house. We must rest at least once when we walk around the block. I may start carrying a fold up chair so she can rest but still get some exercise.

With the new medicine working well I was able to chance a trip to Pacific Grove so she could watch the waves hit the rocks. We picked up a chicken sandwich at McDonald's and parked at a small beach. The ocean was calm, so I took her to the water's edge to sit—not a good idea. A ripple about four or five inches came in, hit her shoes, and splashed her ankles. She stood up, walked forward while trying to turn. In doing so she got wet up to her knees with me hanging onto her arm helping her back to dry land, both of us laughing the whole time. Sonnie would have fallen face forward if I had missed grabbing her arm and I doubt if there would have been any laughter.

I'm going to cut this update off here. I still have some notes to record but there are a few things happening in the next couple of weeks that may prove interesting. You probably will receive another "Sonnie Update" later this month.

- Just me, Steve

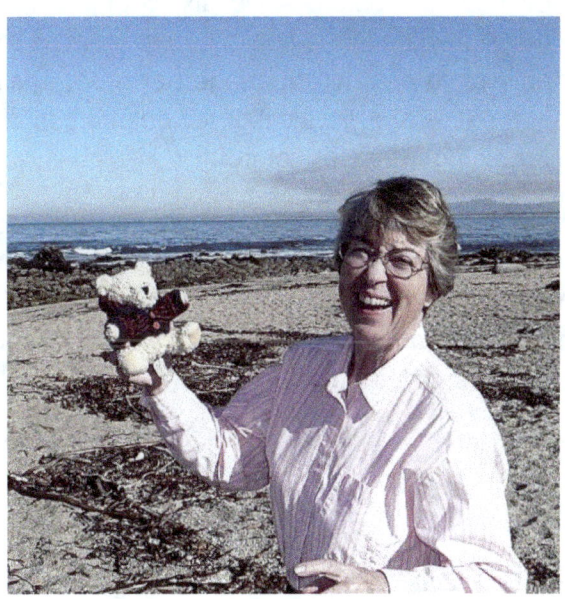

Sonnie and Pee-Wee at the beach
circa 2009

Are The Physical Changes the Alzheimer's or Something Else?

It seemed to happen so quickly that we're not sure if the physical changes Mom was experiencing were due to the Alzheimer's or if she was having small strokes. It seems more likely that she was having small strokes. We don't know and there was no point in taking her into the doctor.

Dad continued to problem solve, fix, change, rig and generally build whatever he could to help Mom be more comfortable or to help him manage her more easily. I think that creative and physical outlet helped him cope. It was something within his control.

I continued to worry about Dad. He was wearing down physically and emotionally. I was seriously considering attempting to talk him into finding a care facility for Mom. But he's a stubborn one, my Daddy. I know he was hiding the worst of it from me.

- Joni

Email Update #16: September 28, 2009

Earlier this year I started to see more physical movement problems with the way Sonnie walked and carried her body. Getting in and out of the car is a challenge for her. I must almost show her what to do and when she does get in, I have to hold her head, so she doesn't bang it on the door frame. When getting out, I must take both hands and help guide her to a standing position and make sure she can stand before letting her go. Her body shakes until she has good footing.

Getting into and out of bed is interesting. She crawls up onto the bed, on her hands and knees, facing across the bed. I must slowly work her into her sleeping position and roll her to her side or back and then she is ready to sleep. When getting out of bed there are times when I must bend her legs at the knees, slide her to the edge of the bed, bring her up to a sitting position, get her feet on the floor, help her to stand up, and wait until she can take her shuffle steps; then away we go.

When getting her dressed I help her back up and lean against the side of the bed with her fanny, then she can lift one foot at a time to put on her underpants and over pants. Otherwise, she can't keep her balance.

I finally changed the doorknob to our bedroom from the locking type to the pass-through type. It got to the point that when she would lock that door, she couldn't remember how to open it and I couldn't open it with the special wire opener while she was trying to open it from the inside. In a couple more years I will have the house remodeled.

I also built handrails for the step that leads into the garage from the family room. I even use them.

I took a class on "Managing Difficult Behavior Without Drugs." I'm not sure it can be done. While I was at the 2-hour class in Monterey, Sonnie was with JoAnn and Joe in Salinas demonstrating "Difficult Behavior With Drugs."

Our dish towels and hand towels are usually pretty clean. I must clean towels once or twice a day. Sonnie not only cleans the counter tops, she will wipe the chairs, the floor anything that she comes in contact with. If you stop by, don't hesitate to ask where we keep the clean towels because you may not know where the one in your hand was last used.

I think I solved a few more problems. I went to "Mattress Discounters" and bought two adjustable extralong twin beds that I can connect and replaced our thirty-plus-year-old king bed. Now I can have my part of the bed raised to help with my Barrett's esophagus, and adjust Sonnie's side to wherever she is comfortable, and be ready for any future needs.

I have two waterproof mattress covers on each bed. Each cover has a fitted sheet over it. After Sonnie has night sweats, I take one fitted sheet and mattress cover off and we're ready for a second night sweat. If there are more, I move her to my side (Joni and I worked that out.)

Sonnie's Journey

While walking with Sonnie around the block earlier this month, she went as far as she could go, and then stopped. No warning. She started to go to the ground; I grabbed her and was helping her to a brick wall to sit on when a man and woman from across the street ran over to lend a hand. They thought she was having a heart attack—I explained the Alzheimer's. The woman ran back, got her car, and gave us a ride home, offering to help in other ways at any time. It's nice to have good neighbors. Now Sonnie starts out by pushing the wheelchair (about 100 yds.) and then gets in it to ride the rest of the way. And yes—she likes to go further now.

Shopping at the store is getting harder as time goes on. Last week at Safeway, we were checking out and Sonnie decided that the "March of Dimes" jar belonged to us and nothing I could say would change her mind. She finally saw everyone staring at us and decided she didn't like the jar anymore.

She weighs about 104 pounds, and she can put her underpants on using any of the three openings. I thought they looked tight, but it took me awhile to figure out that her left leg was through the waist opening.

Our good friend Jerri got me into making smoothies. (Thanks Jerri!) I make at least one every day and put all kinds of goodies in it, including wheat bran, some stuff called Psyllium Husks and of course ice cream. I'm thinking of buying some Pistachios, eating the nuts, and breaking up the shells for her (I'm kidding). Constipation is a problem at times!

About fifteen of you signed up for "Sonnie's Care Plan" last year about this time. Some of you may be unable to continue the list and others may wish to join the list. Let me know so I can update my records. Don't feel badly if you must drop from the list. But feel good if you join the list! I have only had to use a few people so far but as she approaches the last stage of Alzheimer's, I know I will need more help along the way. Even with the new medicine she can still get angry, and it's hard for me to ask anyone to stay with her during these times.

We just got back from a walk and wheelchair ride around the block. It was cool this evening and I put a sweatshirt on Sonnie along with a jacket and gloves. When I was getting her ready for bed, I found that I couldn't get the sweatshirt up over her head and off. It hurts her arms to raise them. I tried several different ways and finally just cut the sweatshirt from the neck down to the waist and it came right off.

She continues to spend an hour or more "going through her mail," looking at the cards (some old) and writing notes or letters and drawing things on the pad of paper I've set out.

More sad news; Sonnie's sister Susie passed away on the 16th of September. Susie and Roger had been fighting her Cancer for the last several years. Sonnie doesn't understand that she is gone but she knows something is wrong. Right now, I feel like Sonnie; I can't find the words I want to say.

I think I'll stop right here. Don't forget to tell your husband or wife, and especially your kids, that you love them. It means a lot!

- Just me, Steve

Her Smiles Are Gone

The last few months were extremely hard. It was so difficult to watch Mom slip farther and farther, faster, and faster, down the spiral.

The Alzheimer's was advancing and effecting not just her voluntary bodily functions but her involuntary functions as well.

She was forgetting how to swallow food.

- Joni

<u>Email Update #17: November 20, 2009</u>

Sonnie's smiles are gone; her facial features are almost always the same. Her eyes are closed a lot of the time and when they are open, they only focus on what she is thinking of or doing. From the beginning of our Journey, we've kept all the greeting cards from friends and family in a box. We call it her mail. She spends a great deal of time "going over her mail," sometimes for hours.

Over the last several months Sonnie's condition has deteriorated at a faster rate. This last month it seems like her condition is in "free fall." She can't really walk anymore and has fallen several times. She received a lot of bruises but only a little blood. No broken bones. Her muscles and joints must give her some pain because she will grimace sometimes when I move her from place to place.

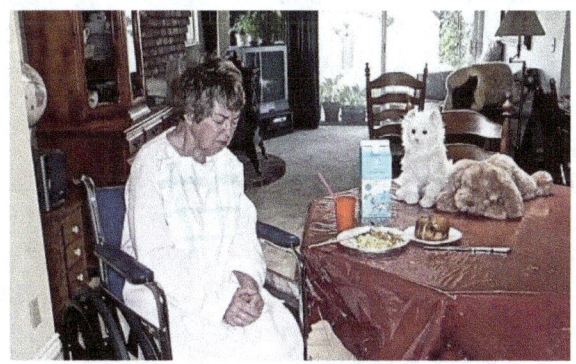

Sonnie November 2009

Sonnie eats most of her meals from the wheelchair. For breakfast I usually feed her myself. There are occasions when I make two or three types of food before she will eat something (oatmeal, cereal, eggs, or maybe hotcakes) but when she eats, she eats well. I make one serving for the two of us, and what she doesn't eat, I eat. She is back down to 100 pounds. I'm down to 163 pounds.

There was one day last month when she had an accident partly in the bed. She was able to get up and make it to the chair when I realized what was happening and she finished in the toilet. She has on protective underpants all the time now.

She doesn't understand brushing her teeth at all. There are times when I get her started brushing in the bathroom and she does well for a while; then she will move the brush from her teeth to the faucet handles and around the sink drain and back to her teeth. Very seldom will she let me help. She loves cinnamon so we mix some in a cup of water and use that as a mouth rinse to freshen her breath.

Going to the toilet is becoming more of a challenge. She is not sure who I am most of the time. She is not about to let me help get her pants down, let alone her underpants. Sometimes when I do talk her into getting her outer pants down, I let her sit on the toilet before I can convince her that her underpants must come down too.

We went to her three-month doctor appointment last week. I'm going to get a handicap sticker for the pickup. It's too hard to get her in and out of the car. I don't know how long I will need it because she is almost to the point where she just wants to stay home. For that matter she sleeps all night and a good part of the day, now.

I read a book last week for the first time in two years. I even have a 1000-piece jigsaw puzzle going.

Now that we use the wheelchair in the house all the time, I guess I will have to have the carpet cleaned by someone who has a bigger machine then I do. It's starting to look pretty bad. We have a metal tack strip dividing the carpet from the tile going into the bathroom from our bedroom. I had to put a scrap piece of carpet over the tack strip. She didn't know what it was and wouldn't step over it.

Joe and I built a ramp into the garage to make it easier to wheel Sonnie around. It came out pretty good.

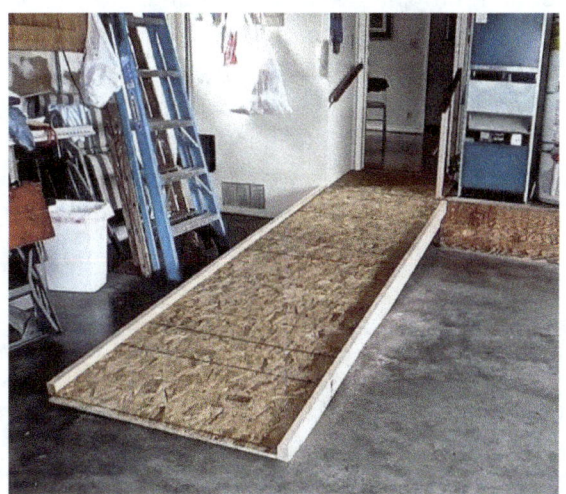

Wheelchair ramp from the garage
Circa November 2009

On October 10th Sonnie started working with her own personal attendant. Adriana is a young woman, probably in her early thirties, and they get along great. We started out with Adriana coming every Wednesday from 12 to 4. Since then, we added Thursday from 12 to 4 and I think it is going to work out fine. She works for Central Coast Seniors, Inc., and I'm pleased with the organization.

I've checked out an assisted living community that has an Alzheimer's and Dementia branch. I have another that I want to check out when Joni is here. I can put a deposit down and hold the next place that becomes available when my name comes to the top of the list. I can just bump my name down one until the time comes (or rather IF the time comes) when I can no longer care for her. My goal is still to keep her with me here at home.

The local Alzheimer's Association asked me to speak for a few minutes at their Annual Memory Walk Rally. Of course, I was just one of many, but it was an honor, and we had a good time. I took Sonnie with me onto the stage and introduced her to the crowd and gave my talk on Alzheimer's and how the Memory Walk would help to someday bring a cure for Alzheimer's. I think that the walk raised something like $85,000. I guess I didn't do too bad, as the Regional Director gave us a thumbs up as we walked off the stage. It seemed like everyone had on a T Shirt that said something about Alzheimer's. If I had a T shirt it would say, "MY WIFE HAS ALZHEIMER'S—BUT SHE DOESN'T KNOW IT" and Sonnie's shirt would say, "I HAVE ALZHEIMER'S AND DON'T YOU FORGET IT." Please, if you're able, donate to the Alzheimer's Association. Thanks!

Since Sonnie needs to be always watched, I made another good investment. I bought a Day and Night Monitor. It has an infrared camera for night vision and a handheld or standalone color video monitor. I use it a lot when Sonnie is napping and I'm in the other room. I'm very happy with the whole thing.

Last month Sonnie was getting these bruises on her upper arms, and it took me the longest time to figure out where they came from. The chairs around our kitchen table are ladder-back chairs. It turns out that she was bumping into the knobs on the top of the chairs. Now I just use folding chairs around the kitchen table.

I've also turned the seat of the chairs we have around the house to the wall; it saves a lot of clean up if she can't make it to the bathroom. That's not so much a problem now because Sonnie can't walk. I can take the double locks off the doors and change all kinds of things back to the way they were if I wanted to. I'll wait a little longer, just in case.

Sonnie's doctor has set it up so I can crush any of her pills and mix them with applesauce or whatever. She does not like to take pills!

It's probably just a sign of the times but her bowel movements only happen about every four to five days. And that's only after I give her a laxative (Senokot – two tablets) on the third and fourth night. Any suggestions?

- Just me, Steve

The End of The Journey

I was lucky enough to be visiting my parents when Mom died.

As hard as it was to lose Mom, it was a blessing that she was finally at the end of her Journey. She was finally at peace.

Rather than return to Phoenix, I sent my family home, and I stayed to help Dad.

The day after Mom died, Dad and I went through the house in Salinas and picked out the very few things he thought he could squeeze into his cabin. One of his dreams in life was to live in his cabin full time. We thought maybe he could do that after Mom was diagnosed with Alzheimer's but her sanctuary, where she was comfortable, was in her Salinas house, so that's where they lived.

Now Dad was ready to move to his sanctuary, the cabin. I stayed for a week. We kept ourselves very busy to put off the grief of losing Mom.

As I am finding as I write this book for Dad, it turns out that my compartmentalizing is not a very healthy grief strategy. After Mom died, I wouldn't allow myself to cry. On the flight back to Phoenix, as the tears threatened, I ruthlessly pushed them back. Not a very healthy coping mechanism, but that's me. I was afraid to cry. I was afraid that if I let myself cry, I would never stop. It was 11 months later that the dam finally burst. I was in my car alone, on the way to the mall to go Christmas shopping when I simply started to sob uncontrollably. I pulled off the road into an empty parking lot and let the tears come.

Grieving is a process. You can't run from it, hide from it, or avoid it. You must go through it. Oh well; maybe now I will finally allow myself the time to grieve and heal.

Like Daddy, I think of Mommy every day. I keep reminders of her all around me.

I miss her.

- Joni

Email Update #18: January 19, 2010

It's hard to believe that Sonnie has been gone for 19 days. This will be the last group email update I send out. Don't feel obligated to answer it. Most of you have already sent a card or contacted me in other ways. I won't be answering all the cards and emails because there are so many of them and I'm not very good at it anyway. But I do want to thank everyone for being my support group and taking this Journey with us.

Writing this is going to be harder than I thought—tears are already filling my eyes.

During December we seldom left the house. Getting Sonnie into the pickup truck to go for a ride got to be scary for her and a chore for me. It was so hard to get her into the truck that I was afraid if I took her out in the wheelchair into a store, I wouldn't be able to get her back in the truck after shopping.

It got to where Sonnie was sleeping sixteen to twenty hours a day, and I would have trouble waking her to feed her. Sometimes it would take me twenty minutes to wake her. Toward the end she would keep her eyes closed about 90% of the time when she was awake. I could see her eyes moving under her lids, but I think she was afraid of the things she would see, particularly if there were other people around or busy sounds.

For the last three or four weeks, I cut half inch strips of plywood at different lengths, wrapped them with towels and placed them on the right side of her wheelchair just to keep her shoulders and head from listing too far to the right. They worked pretty well; I was able to feed her easier and she looked more comfortable.

In early December, the pastor from her church came by and gave her communion in our home. Then again, just before Christmas, he came by with a women's group called "The Circle of Joy" and they sang Christmas Carols for us. Jake and his family were with us. A couple times when they would finish a song Sonnie would raise her hands a few inches from her lap and clap (the tears are back). They were very dainty claps, but they were claps.

Joni and her family came out on the 29th of December. They stayed at our cabin at night, and we would see them during the day. Joni was the last person able to feed Sonnie any amount of food at all on the evening of the 31st. Sonnie was to the point where she would have trouble swallowing food or liquids and would hold most foods in her cheeks and even along her gum lines.

January 1st started out like I expected. I got Sonnie up and on the potty chair then put her on a small computer chair with wheels, rolled her into the bathroom and gave her a bath-shower. After getting her dressed she had just a little breakfast of oatmeal and fruit and then she was ready to go back to sleep. I don't remember the time, but I had her sleep on the couch in the family room because I had a small fire going in the wood stove and the temperature seemed about right.

It was around noon when I woke her up for lunch. I put her in her wheelchair and rolled her to the bedroom for another trip to the potty chair— I'll stop here and just say that there was no indication of discomfort or stress except for a split second when her heart attack struck. I called 911 when I realized she was having a heart attack. Then I called Joni and told her Mom was having a heart attack. By the time she ran over to get my son Jake and start driving into town, Sonnie had died.

I think I need to make this suggestion to anyone that may read Sonnie's Journey. Go out today or tomorrow, no later than the next day, and start the paperwork for a Living Trust. Get a good attorney and make sure the trust contains a Will, an Advanced Health Care Directive and a Directive for Personal Property and Power of Attorney. For Sonnie, we also had a Do Not Resuscitate (DNR) order.

I needed the DNR to stop the paramedics from doing chest compressions and let her pass.

Death Certificate: Cardiopulmonary Arrest. Underlying Cause: Alzheimer's Disease.

Epilogue

In October of 2010, I spoke again at the Alzheimer's Association Annual Memory Walk Rally.

Sonnie wasn't with me, I took an empty wheelchair.

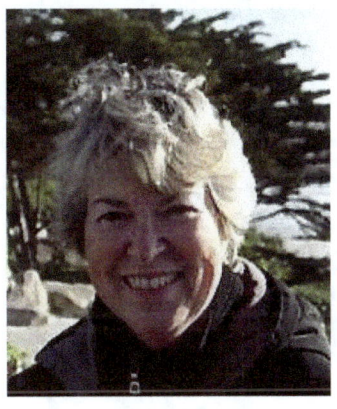

Sondra Jo (Herrick) Goetz
Salinas

Sondra Jo (Herrick) Goetz, know to those who loved her as Sonnie, died at home on January 1, 2010 at the age of 70 after a long Journey with Alzheimer's. Sonnie was born in Albion, Michigan on September 14, 1939 where she lived until a vacation to California in 1961. She made it as far as Carmel on that vacation, decided to stay and soon thereafter met her husband, Steve Goetz. Steve and Sonnie married in 1962 and have two children, Jake and Joni; 4 grandchildren, Jessica, Zachary, Jake and Clint; and four great-grandchildren, Drew, Logan, Ronin and Riley. There were no services as Sonnie dreaded funerals. A Celebration of Life was held for family and friends a few months after her death. Should you wish to honor Sonnie's memory, please donate to the Alzheimer's Association.

Life Goes On

Daddy was so lonely after Mom died. He had dedicated six years to taking care of her and grieving her loss slowly as he watched her die. She had the best of care.

I was thrilled the day Dad called to tell me he started reaching out to old friends. He wanted to reconnect after being isolated taking care of Mom. I told him, "You have a great big heart and there is plenty of room in there for everyone." I know that finding love again in his life didn't make him love my mom any less.

I also know that having a loving companion in the later years of life will keep him alive years longer than anything I can do for him. Too many times you hear about people who lose parents within a year or two of each other. I believe they die from loneliness.

Getting out and living life, every day, is what's important. None of us know how much time we have on this earth. We all need to make the most of each and every day with love in our hearts for everyone who has gone before us and be present with those we have in our life to love today.

- Joni

Steve Update #1: March 15, 2020

Sonnie has been gone now for over 10 years.

When I was a kid, I preferred to be alone. I spent many days at my grandmother's home in the Palo Colorado Canyon roaming the hills. After being married to Sonnie, I realized how important having someone to love and love me back was for my life.

As Sonnie's Alzheimer's advanced, she became less and less comfortable around people. We became isolated from our friends.

Shortly after Sonnie passed away, I made plans to visit with everyone who was on my Care Plan to thank them for helping or being willing to help.

First on my list was Ginger. She was the widow of one of my very best friend Ron. Ron had passed in 2003 from a brain tumor. I called to make arrangements to stop by and visit a while. After that we started dating and were together for almost 9 years. We both enjoyed flowers, national parks, and lots of other things. Toward the end of the summer in 2019, we decided to take separate paths, but are still very close friends.

Joni came for one of her visits in mid-October of 2019. We decided to call up a few of Mom's other good friends and go out to dinner. JoAnn was Sonnie's very dear friend, and her husband became one of my best friends as well. Joe passed from cancer in 2016. JoAnn and I have been dating ever since.

Reconnecting with good friends is important. There is shared history which makes that friendship very deep and strong, a great foundation for companionship and love.

There's not a day that goes by that I don't think of Sonnie. I have a picture of her and Smoky, her dog, in my bedroom. Reminders of her are everywhere. She is part of me and fortunately my friends feel the same way. Their husbands are still a part of them. We talk of old times together often.

...life is good.

- Just me, Steve